D0684228

My Dream to Trample AIDS:

What everyone at any age
should know about HIV/AIDS

Don Carrel

© 2011 Carrel Care LLC
All Rights Reserved.

No part of this publication may be reproduced, stored in a retrieval system, or transmitted, in any form or by any means, electronic, mechanical, photocopying, recording, or otherwise, without the written permission of the author.

First published by Dog Ear Publishing
4010 W. 86th Street, Ste H
Indianapolis, IN 46268
www.dogearpublishing.net

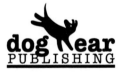

dog ear
PUBLISHING

ISBN: 978-145750-672-7

This book is printed on acid-free paper.

Printed in the United States of America

This book is dedicated to my sons, Chris and Matt,
who gave me a reason to survive the
first 10 years of my life with HIV

and

To my best friend, Dennis,
and my "kid brother," Kenny,
who did not survive,
but will be remembered forever

and

To my partner in life, Chris Curry,
who has been a continual source of love and support
for the last 15 years of my life with AIDS

Contents

Foreword

Every semester my students get an assignment to write a letter to Don Carrel. Who is Don Carrel? Why would you write a letter to him? And why should you care? Don is a man whom I've come to know both professionally and personally through his HIV-positive status. Funny to say that you met someone this way, but as a high-school teacher, we're always looking for guest speakers to present on health topics to our sophomore, co-ed Health & Wellness classes. You might call it education. You might call it "edu-tain-ment." You might call it career exploration depending on the exper-tise and background of the speaker. In Don's case, it's a wake-up call to the teens in my area, a place we fondly refer to as the "Golden Ghetto," where kids are untouchable.

Don gets to teens in a way that the everyday, familiar, "know-it-all" classroom teacher cannot. Try as I might, with humorous sto-ries, outlandish clothing, amazing statistics, riveting film clips, or scintillating current events, I cannot replicate the way Don holds them spellbound. He gets to them, this quiet-spoken man who speaks from experience. Not only is Don HIV-positive and has been since the early 1980's, he has full-blown AIDS. He has lived the major portion of his life under the cloud of his "status."

I first met Don in 1996. We have similar backgrounds – Shawnee Mission Schools, suburbs of Kansas City. He's a few years older. He used to speak to our individual health classes, sometimes five or six presentations in a day – pretty hard on any-one, even the professional teacher. That was tough on his health and also involved the giving up of many workdays on his part. He was a businessman at the time, running *Kids Plus,* a children's toy store. At some point, a 50-minute class segment was just not enough time, so we expanded the presentation to a block day – closer to 85 minutes, which allows Don time to do the topic justice, in his own way. We schedule it as an in-house field trip each semes-ter for all the health sections at once.

During his presentation Don tells his adult life story. He relates tales of others with HIV/AIDS who were his friends or acquaintances and what their relationship meant to him. He passes around containers of pills and other medicines that are expensive daily regimens for AIDS patients. He provides a handout of pertinent U.S. and worldwide AIDS statistics, including local HIV testing information. At the conclusion, he invites students to ask questions. The students sit in rapt attention, with no chatting, goofing around or checking of cell phones. It's a sight to behold. He doesn't speak down to them. He doesn't judge. He doesn't preach.

At this point in the semester, the health students are fairly well read on a variety of health topics and are comfortable asking questions about what may be seen as "touchy" issues. They are also intelligent enough to know there are questions that need to be asked about all of the topics we cover and that **not** knowing (i.e. ignorance) can indeed kill you or negatively influence your health. With HIV/AIDS transmission, the obvious risk factors are the use of IV drugs, unprotected sexual activity and blood-to-blood contact. Some might say high-school students shouldn't be using drugs and/or having sexual relations. In utopia that might be true. But in reality, drugs and sexuality are either in their present or the possibility/probability is in their near future. Teens can be notoriously reckless with their actions and choices.

Don amazingly connects with them not as the grandfather he is, but as a person who was infected before we knew much at all about HIV and even less about HIV transmission. He is grateful for the fact that he was infected before anyone knew better. But today's students **do know** better. After the students hear Don's story, if they subsequently become infected by their own actions or lack of action, they were just not paying attention.

As a follow-up to Don's presentation, students are assigned to write a letter to Don. In their letters, the students tell him at least one new thing they learned about HIV/AIDS. They tell him what impacted them the most about his presentation. They often share unsolicited details with him of the current state of teenage drug use and sexual activity. They also give him feedback about how he could improve his presentation, and he invites them to contact him via email if they have any further questions or concerns. These communications are all confidential. He often shares anonymous anecdotes from students, which are relatable to our own, in later presentations. The letters also have helped provide Don with some of the material for this book.

We know so much more about HIV/AIDS than we used to and are open about discussing the modes of transmission. The fewer students that get infected by HIV, the greater the probability is of a longer and better quality of life for those students. The fewer HIV infections, the less the burden is on the health-care system and a family's finances. Most important, the fewer HIV infections, the less heartache there will be for family, friends and lovers. Don is changing students' lives and forcing them to face the reality of the consequences of their decisions in a way that I cannot. He feels that this is his purpose and is why he has greatly outlived his diagnosis.

> Peggy Rose
> Health Educator
> Blue Valley High School
> Stilwell, Kansas

Introduction

It amazes me how one dream has changed the entire course of my life. In 1995, when I had a dream not suggesting but telling me that I was going to help prevent others from being infected with HIV, I never imagined what would follow. Since that dream, I've had the chance to share my story with more than 100,000 teenagers and adults.

When I started sharing my story, I wasn't an accomplished public speaker. Quite the contrary, I had always been terrified to speak to even small groups of people. Before I ever began my journey to educate others, I expressed my fear of speaking publicly to a friend. He touched his heart and said, *"Don, just remember to speak from here."* Then he touched his forehead and said, *"And not from here."*

I knew how it felt to have AIDS – and how it felt to watch people I loved die from the disease. Talking from my heart about my feelings, rather than concentrating on giving out facts and figures made a lot of sense. Something inside clicked. I suddenly realized I could conquer my fear of speaking if I just took my friend's advice.

I would like to thank the thousands of teenagers and young adults who, over the years, have helped me improve my story by evaluating my presentation and providing me with their own stories to share.

As you read this book you will see numerous quotes. They are in **bold print** and *italics*. These quotes are from teenagers who have taken the time to write me. As you read these quotes, keep in mind that they are from high school students who are typically freshmen and sophomores – ages 14, 15 and 16. I have taken the liberty to "improve" the spelling and grammar as needed in these quotations.

When I speak, I have a habit of "spilling my guts," and students often spill theirs in return. Letters frequently include very personal and specific details about past sexual encounters. Times seem to have changed since I was a teen in the 1960s. I'm convinced that teenagers today are more sexually active than they were in my day. They definitely are more comfortable talking about sex than my peers and I were when we were in high school.

I have accumulated hundreds of personal stories from teens, and I've shared them with others. It is common for a letter to include details about sex, drug use and experience with alcohol, details I'm sure most would never share with their parents or teachers. Years ago, I was shocked with some of the things they wrote. For example, the first time a 15-year-old told me she couldn't remember how many sex partners she had been involved with, I was dumbfounded. Since then, I've heard the same thing from a number of young teens, both male and female. I'm rarely shocked today.

"Don ...Listening to you made me realize how many of my friends are in danger. My best friend lost her virginity when she was only 12 years old. She's now 16 and has sex all the time with her boyfriends, and she has a new boyfriend at least once a week. I'm scared for her." – Elizabeth

"Hi Don ... My best friend just turned 18. She has had at least 30 partners since the age of 12. She rarely thinks of using condoms or any other form of contraceptives." – Danielle

As my presentation has improved, so has my impact on those hearing it. However, over the years, I have become increasingly frustrated. The more people I've been able to share my story with, the more I realize how many people, of all ages, are not aware they are at risk of contracting HIV. They are not aware of how the disease affects every aspect of their daily life physically, financially and emotionally. When someone truly understands all the issues those with HIV/AIDS deal with daily, a person is much more likely to take the steps needed to prevent infection.

I've been HIV-positive since 1981 and have had full-blown AIDS since 1995. Sadly, only about 2 percent or less of those infected with HIV the year I was are still living. I'm blessed, and lucky to be here. I have come to **know** that one of the main reasons I'm still here is because God wants me to tell my story to others. When I was diagnosed, I was told to expect to die within two years – by age 38. Now as I enter my 60s, it's almost unbelievable to think I might actually die of "old age" and not from complications of AIDS.

"Don … I thank God for giving you this disease, but keeping you alive, so that you may teach us what we all need to know to stay alive and well. By coming and speaking to groups of kids, I guarantee that you save <u>many</u> lives, mine is probably one of them." – Alex

"Don … I know that you will have a great life through your disease because God is using you to help people. God will never let you leave before you fulfill your purpose in life and that's what I believe you are doing. I hope that more young people will be greatly moved by your teaching like I was." – Anita

"Dear Don … First of all let me tell you how brave you are to stand up in front of thousands and thousands of teens and tell them about your personal struggle with AIDS. I believe that God has you here for a mission and he won't bring you home until He believes that you have completed that mission successfully." – Tasha

After hearing my story, many teenagers have told me I should *"talk to the entire school … should talk to more schools … that everyone needs to hear my story."*

"Dear Don … PLEASE keep up the good work and continue teaching teenagers. <u>Just</u> a suggestion, once you've gone to all the schools around here, move on to the rest of the country." – Anita

"Dear Don … In my opinion, every school everywhere should hear about your life and what you have been through. You have made me more self conscious about the decisions I will make in my life. … If I'm ever in a position of risk, I will ask myself, 'What would Don do?'" – Danny

I'm taking the advice of Anita, Danny and hundreds of others who have heard my story and I'm taking my message *"to the rest of the country"* and possibly, to the world. Many years of my life have been devoted to teaching others the steps they can easily take to prevent HIV and avoid this dreadful disease.

However, I'm only one person. I'm now a grandfather and I won't be around forever. It is my sincere hope that by writing this book, along with the help of my many teenage friends, I can continue to tell my story long after I'm gone.

CHAPTER 1

My Dream

One morning in September 1995, I was working at *Kids Plus* as I had done most mornings since first opening up the toy and gift store. After working for only a couple of hours, I was exhausted to the point I was barely able to walk and felt worse than I could ever remember. Including my mother, Shirley, there were three of us working at *Kids Plus* that morning. Before lunch, I told Mom I felt horrible and needed to leave for the day.

When I arrived home, I parked in the garage and struggled from the car through the door into my family room and collapsed, too tired to attempt even a trip to the bedroom. I woke up on the sofa later that afternoon with a fever of 105. Before nightfall, I was in the emergency room of Saint Luke's Hospital in Kansas City, Missouri.

After running a few tests, the doctor walked into my hospital room to deliver the news I was dreading. I had Pneumocystis carinii pneumonia, commonly known as PCP, the most frequent cause of death for people with AIDS. My CD4 count was zero, meaning my immune system was no longer functioning.

I had been diagnosed with HIV nine years earlier, but my health had been excellent, until just the last few months. I knew that having PCP meant I was no longer just a person infected with HIV; I had just progressed to someone living with full-blown AIDS.

As I lay in the hospital, I was not afraid of dying. In fact, I was "ready to go." During the last nine years, I had emotionally come to grips with the fact that I would die from complications of AIDS.

I was in a reflective, almost cheerful mood. God had answered my prayers by giving me almost a decade of good health so that I could raise my sons, Chris and Matt. They were only 11 and 8, respectively, when I first learned I was HIV-positive. Yes, I had been extremely lucky. A number of friends and acquaintances who had been diagnosed with HIV around the same time had passed away years before.

One night while I was asleep in the hospital, I had a dream. In my dream, I felt as if I were floating in a huge, puffy white cloud drifting slowly through a perfectly blue sky. Even though I was alone, I felt protected and loved. Suddenly, I heard a forceful, yet gentle, voice say to me, *"Don, I'm sorry, but you're not going to die now. You still have a job to do. You're going to go out and teach teenagers what they need to know so that they never get AIDS."*

I woke up immediately. It had been a short dream, but I knew instantly my life was going to change. I was going to leave the hospital. I was not going to die anytime soon. I somehow understood the messenger in my dream did not intend for me to talk to simply a few teenagers. I sensed I would be talking to hundreds and hundreds of them.

I was bewildered by this new knowledge as well as quite angry. Over the previous six months, I had started to lose weight, and my health and energy level had deteriorated significantly. Once I finally managed to drag myself out of bed each morning, I would head to the bathroom to shave. After shaving, I was so exhausted that I had to lie down for a while before I had the energy to shower. After showering, I would lie down again to rest until I finally had enough energy to get dressed.

Life was no longer any fun. It had become a complete struggle, and I had lost any desire to live. I was emotionally and physically ready to die. How in the world was I supposed to teach thousands of teenagers and young adults about HIV/AIDS when I could barely dress myself in the morning?

I had no interest in going out in the world and talking to people about AIDS. Not only was I convinced I couldn't handle it physically, I was terrified of the prospect of *any* kind of public speaking.

Despite my anger and fear, I somehow knew I had no choice in the matter. It was fact; I was going to tell my story to teens and adults in order to help prevent them from contracting HIV. And yet, I had no idea how to get started.

Two weeks after my PCP diagnosis, I was discharged from the hospital, sitting in a wheelchair, unable to walk and hooked up to an oxygen tank. Even though I was nearly six feet tall, I weighed only 119 pounds. I looked as if I had just been released from a concentration camp. I lay at home for months, slowly recovering and thinking about my dream each day. Weeks passed, and I still had no idea how I would ever be able to accomplish my mission.

Apparently, "the messenger" in my dream had a plan, and it must have worked. Since that night, I've had the chance to share my story with more than 100,000 teenagers and adults. That dream changed the entire course of my life. It may be hard to fathom, but during my incredible journey of the last 15 years, I've come to believe that having HIV is a huge *blessing* in my life. As you read my story, I hope you will begin to understand why.

CHAPTER 2
HIV and AIDS – The Basics

I hope that after reading this book you will have a greater understanding about how HIV/AIDS has affected my life, the lives of many of my friends and how contracting HIV would affect your life. Thousands of teenagers and adults have told me that before hearing my presentation they had a basic understanding that having HIV/AIDS would require them to take medication and could eventually lead to death. However, hearing my story helped them understand what it would actually *"feel like to have the disease."* After learning what the daily struggles of living with the disease entailed, they *"don't want to ever contract HIV."* As you read you will start to understand why dying from complications of AIDS is far easier than living day after day with the consequences of having HIV.

Experience has taught me that those who understand how HIV/AIDS impacts everyday life while they are still living are much more likely to practice safer sex or abstain from premarital sex altogether. They're also more likely to avoid the use of any drugs, which might potentially lead to intravenous drug use.

With that in mind, I'm first going to cover some basic information about HIV/AIDS, and the manner in which the virus is transmitted.

Acquired Immune Deficiency Syndrome (AIDS) is a disease of the immune system caused by the Human Immunodeficiency Virus (HIV). Many people who contract HIV have no physical symptoms at the time they are initially infected. Some who are infected experience "seroconversion" illnesses, which can include one or more of the following: flu-like symptoms, fever, nausea, diarrhea, sore throat, mouth ulcers, rashes, aching muscles and swollen lymph nodes. These symptoms generally present themselves between two and six weeks after infection. In most cases, seroconversion illnesses only last for a day or two and are not severe enough to warrant a visit to the doctor. However, in a few cases, the illnesses are more severe and may last up to six months.

When someone is infected with HIV, his or her immune system starts to deteriorate. HIV attacks a type of infection fighting white blood cell in the immune system known as a T-cell. As a result, the number of T-cells decrease, which causes the lowering of someone's T-cell "count" (commonly called a CD4 count).

For example, prior to becoming infected with HIV, a healthy individual might have a CD4 count of 1,100. Once infected, this 1,100 CD4 count starts to decrease gradually. As the CD4 count decreases, the body's ability to fight off infection also decreases. Once the CD4 count has reached somewhere between 200 and 300, the immune system is seriously damaged, and the person is likely to develop various infections and cancers that may result in death.

The difference between having HIV and having AIDS is determined by the progression of the disease and the amount of immune system damage. Once the CD4 count of someone infected with HIV has decreased to 200 or below, it's very likely the individual will develop an **opportunistic infection**. An opportunistic infection is an acute condition that can end in death; an example is Pneumocystis carinii pneumonia (PCP). Once someone infected with HIV has a CD4 count of 200 or below and develops an opportunistic infection, he or she has AIDS.

Once infected with HIV, it used to take an average of eight to 12 years for most people to progress to AIDS. In my case, it took 15 years. However, since the introduction of more effective HIV medications in the mid-1990s, it now often takes much longer for people with HIV to progress to full-blown AIDS. This means that with proper care, those newly infected with the virus can expect to remain healthier for a much longer period. The implications of developing AIDS have also changed. AIDS was once considered a fatal illness. Today, living with HIV/AIDS is similar to living with other chronic diseases such as diabetes. Thanks to improvements in treatment, those living with HIV/AIDS today may actually die from old age, something that has nothing to do with their HIV infection.

Americans first began dying from the effects of AIDS in 1980. Initially, public health officials did not know AIDS was caused by a virus and weren't sure of all the ways the disease could be transmitted from one person to another. It was 1984 before HIV was actually identified and 1985 before an HIV test was available to determine if someone was infected.

Early in the AIDS epidemic, people were terrified to be around anyone with this "new fatal disease." It was common for people to assume that AIDS could be transmitted as easily as the common cold. Many people believe it was possible to contract the disease if an infected person sneezed or coughed on them or they drank out of the same glass, shared a fork or even happened to be in the same room. People were terrified to be in the presence of anyone with AIDS.

We now know that AIDS is not transmitted as easily as the common cold. None of the above examples transmits the virus.

HIV can be found in levels sufficient to infect others in the following four body fluids:

- **Blood**

- **Semen**

- **Vaginal Fluid**

- **Breast Milk**

To contract HIV, the virus must enter a person's blood stream. Any activity that could put an infected person's blood, semen or vaginal fluid into the blood stream of another individual can result in infection with HIV. HIV enters the body through open cuts; sores; breaks in the skin; mucous membranes, such as those inside the anus or vagina or direct injection. If you understand these facts, you are well on your way to understanding what precautions you must take to minimize your risk of ever contracting HIV/AIDS.

Today, nearly all HIV infections in the United States occur because of sexual contact or sharing needles, syringes or other injection equipment with someone who is infected.

Prior to the introduction of newer, more effective HIV drugs in the mid 1990s, it was common for an HIV-positive mother to transmit the disease to her unborn child. However, it's now known that pregnant women with HIV who take HIV medication during their pregnancy, deliver their child by C-section and do not breast-feed their babies (HIV can pass from mother to child in breast milk) reduce the risk of passing the virus on to the baby to 2 percent or less.

Contracting HIV from a blood transfusion or blood products was common in the early 1980s during the beginning of the AIDS epidemic, but is rare today because most countries now screen blood for HIV antibodies prior to use.

Since the beginning of the HIV/AIDS epidemic, possible routes of transmission have been thoroughly investigated by state and local health departments and the Centers for Disease Control. HIV has been detected in saliva, tears and urine. However, the concentration of HIV in these fluids is low and there has never been a single reported case of HIV transmission through these fluids.

HIV cannot be transmitted through day-to-day activities such as shaking hands or kissing. You also cannot become infected from a mosquito bite, toilet seat, drinking fountain, or sharing food or eating utensils with someone who is HIV-positive.

CHAPTER 3
About Don

Since I began my crusade to help prevent others from contracting HIV/AIDS, I've had the privilege of telling my story to thousands of people of all ages. When I first started, I talked to small groups and did not have a "canned" presentation containing a lot of facts and figures. Instead, I had a conversation with others about how HIV had affected my life and the lives of a few of my close friends. Over the years, I've answered many questions and learned from experience what basic information most people would like to know about HIV/AIDS.

While I continue to concentrate on talking from my heart about the personal and emotional impact of the disease, I've learned to incorporate the answers to commonly asked questions into my presentation. I have no prepared speech; however, I have an outline I normally follow.

If you were sitting in an audience about to hear my presentation, here is how it would typically begin:

Hi – My name is Don Carrel, but please call me "Don." Before I get started, I would like to give you a quick outline of what I'm going to talk about today. My presentation is in six parts.

- *First, I'm going to tell you a little bit about myself.*

- *Second, I'm going to tell you about a couple of friends of mine who had HIV and describe the impact this disease had on their lives.*

- *Third, I'm going to talk about the history of HIV/AIDS and discuss some HIV/AIDS statistics.*

- *Fourth, I'm going to talk about HIV testing and who in this room should consider being tested for HIV.*

• Fifth, I'll talk about what medication and treatment is available for those with HIV/AIDS.

• Finally, I'm going to give you some information about what steps you can take to help make sure you never end up like me – a person living with AIDS.

When I am finished speaking, I'll be more than happy to answer questions. It's my policy to answer any question that someone asks, provided I know the answer. If you have a personal question you would like to ask me, and you're not comfortable doing so in public, you're welcome to call or e-mail me.

I would like to begin by telling you a little about myself. I grew up in Shawnee, Kansas, a suburb of Kansas City. I graduated from Shawnee Mission North High School and then obtained my bachelor's degree from Kansas State University in Manhattan, Kansas. Shortly after graduating from K-State, I married and within five years, my wife and I had two sons, Christopher and Matthew.

My wife and I divorced when Chris and Matt were four and one. After my divorce, I started dating again. It wasn't long after I started dating that I became infected with HIV, the virus that causes AIDS.

To the best of my knowledge, I was infected with HIV in 1981. Believe it or not, I'm glad I was infected then because in 1981, no one knew about HIV. It was 1980 when four Americans, the first of many, died of AIDS, but it was 1984 before scientists finally discovered HIV. Since HIV was unheard of in 1981, no one, including me, was warned about catching it. As a result, I never have felt guilty or personally responsible for catching HIV. I wasn't careless. I didn't know any better.

Coping with the emotional, physical and financial aspects of having HIV/AIDS is difficult. The fact I'm HIV-positive is on my mind almost every hour of every day. Dealing with having this disease is hard enough. I'm very thankful I don't also have to deal with feeling as if it was my fault for catching it. In 1981, I had no idea my sexual behavior was putting me at risk for contracting a fatal disease.

You, on the other hand, have grown up knowing HIV/AIDS is out there, waiting for anyone who is careless enough to catch it. If you put yourself at risk for HIV and end up with the disease, you'll not only have to cope with having HIV, you also will have to live with the *fact that it is your fault you are infected. You should have known better.*

Even though I believe I was infected with HIV in 1981, I didn't know for sure until I had an HIV test in September 1986. I'll never forget the day the doctor gave me my test results. Dr. Wade walked into the room and said, "Don, I'm sorry to have to tell you, but you do have the virus that causes AIDS ... I suggest you get your affairs in order. Based on what we know about this disease today, you'll be sick within a year and will more than likely die within two."

Obviously, my doctor was wrong. It has been 25 years since I was matter-of-factly informed I would die within two years. Yet I'm still here. However, I had four friends who tested HIV-positive about the same time I did. All four of them were given the same two-year "death sentence" by their doctor. Over the next two to three years, I watched in horror as all four of them got sick – and then sicker – and finally died. In the mid-1980s, there was no medication available to treat anyone with HIV/AIDS and as a result, most people diagnosed with AIDS did die within a couple of years.

I had no physical symptoms of this disease for the first 14 years I was infected. From 1981 until 1995, I was completely healthy. I felt fine. As far as I can remember, I never had the flu or any other illness that kept me home from work during all those years. I don't even remember having a cold. Starting in the summer of 1995, however, my health began deteriorating rapidly. Six months later, I was hospitalized with Pneumocystis carinii pneumonia, commonly called PCP. PCP is the most common cause of death for someone with AIDS. Amazingly, I survived. When I was released from the hospital, even though I was nearly six feet tall, I weighed only 119 pounds, which is 61 pounds less than my current weight. My CD4 count was zero. A CD4 count is a measurement of how well your immune system is working. An average healthy young adult might have a CD4 count of approximately 1100. A zero CD4 count indicated my immune system was not working. I no longer just had HIV. I now had AIDS.

When I speak, I always point out that I'm not just HIV-positive; I have full-blown AIDS. However, no one can tell I have AIDS from my appearance. Even though I have had HIV for almost 30 years, I look completely healthy. Before today, if you thought you would be able to tell someone was infected because he or she would look "sick," I should be all the proof you need to know that you cannot tell if someone is infected with HIV from their appearance.

"Don ... You are the first person I've ever actually met or seen in person with AIDS and you are living proof that just because someone has AIDS it doesn't mean that they'll 'look' unhealthy." – Trey

"Don ... You look like you are perfectly fine to me, but I guess that's what's dangerous about it." – Nick

"Dear Don ... I thought it was a great idea for a person who actually has AIDS to come and speak. They usually give us the boring normal lecture, but you actually know what happens with AIDS. ... It makes me sad to know that so much of your life has been impacted by one disease." – Brent

"Don ... Before you spoke I had the average 'It won't happen to me' attitude. I thought, 'How many people do I actually know that have AIDS?' But now I realize that I might be faced with a lot of people who have AIDS or are HIV-positive. I now realize that these people don't wear a sign that says 'I have AIDS.' Now I know that they walk, eat, drink just like everybody else." – Ashley

"Dear Don ... Wow, where do I start ... I sincerely knew that AIDS and HIV were very common, but I'd never been in the same room with someone who had it. I honestly had a preconceived idea of what you would look like. ... I pictured a sickly, frail man but you look great!" – Emily

"Dear Don ... I walked into the classroom on Wednesday thinking I would hear a boring lecture on safe sex. I walked out of the room knowing I had learned much more. You are a person that knows how to get through to students. You don't just give the facts you live them." – Jeremy

"Dear Don ... When you came to speak to my class about AIDS, it greatly impacted my life. You really made me understand what it would feel like to be an AIDS patient. ... I just sat there astounded the whole time and I kept thinking of what it would feel and be like to have it. ... If I had AIDS, I would just be a hermit at home and would not make good use of the situation, like you do. I'd also like to congratulate you on being so courageous and brave to stand up in front of a group of teasing, inconsiderate teenagers and tell the things you've done." – Mark

CHAPTER 4

My "Best Friend" – Dennis

My best friend, Dennis, was the first person I knew with HIV. When I met Dennis in the early 1980s, he was about 35, a doctor of veterinary medicine, a specialist in rabies research and a member of the faculty at Kansas State University. Early in our friendship, we formed the habit of meeting for lunch every Wednesday. One Wednesday, in March 1986, I met Dennis at *The Hibachi Hut*, where we often had lunch. In the middle of lunch, out of the blue, Dennis looked at me and said, *"Don, I have something I need to tell you … I just found out I have AIDS."* I was devastated. Dennis was my best friend. I instantly understood that Dennis had just told me he was going to die.

Up until lunch that day, I knew people were being diagnosed with HIV/AIDS and dying, but at that point in time, most of the infections appeared to be either on the East Coast in New York City or on the West Coast in San Francisco. I had never heard of a single person in the Midwest with HIV. How could Dennis, who was living in Manhattan, Kansas, a college town in the middle of the country, have a disease that only appeared to infect people living on the coasts?

I was in tears within seconds after learning my closest friend had HIV. Dennis, on the other hand, did not appear to be the least bit concerned. The "physician" in him was doing the talking. He continued, *"There's nothing I can do about it now. So far, I feel fine. I'm going to continue to go to work every day, teach my classes and do my research. I'm not going to worry about it until I get sick and can't take care of myself. When that happens … I'm going to commit suicide."*

When Dennis told me he was going to commit suicide, I believed him. One day I was in his office while he was treating a dog. The poor pup was in considerable pain and there was nothing Dennis could do to stop the suffering or save the dog's life. I watched him slowly fill a syringe, sit down and pick up the dog. He held his patient gently in his lap and slowly injected the drug into a vein. The dog laid his head on Dennis' arm and closed his eyes for the last time. As a doctor, Dennis had the knowledge and means to "put himself to sleep." I was convinced he'd do so once his HIV progressed to full-blown AIDS and he could no longer lead a normal, productive life.

However, Dennis never committed suicide. He never took his own life because he was mentally incapable of doing so. He developed the worse case of AIDS-related dementia I've ever seen. The symptoms of AIDS-related dementia are similar to those of Alzheimer's; the ability to think rationally is seriously affected. AIDS-related dementia is quite common and almost everyone I've known with AIDS developed dementia at some point before death. However, in most cases the dementia is fairly mild until the last few days or weeks of life. Dennis had a case of early onset dementia. He lost the ability to think rationally many months before he started to deteriorate physically.

Dennis was extremely intelligent, a brilliant researcher and a well-respected professor. As a doctor of pathology, he was involved in a number of groundbreaking studies at K-State. About a year after being diagnosed with HIV, it became apparent that his ability to think clearly was starting to be affected. At first, he reminded me of someone in the early stages of Alzheimer's. One minute he would seem perfectly normal and then the next he might say or do something completely insane.

For example, one day Dennis did some grocery shopping. He filled his cart full of food, and when he finished shopping, he pushed the cart out the door, but never went through the checkout to pay for his groceries. While Dennis was loading food into his trunk, the police arrived.

At the time, I owned a retail store and café next door to the grocery store. One of my employees rushed into my office to tell me she saw a police car arrive with its lights flashing and that two officers got out of the car and were talking to Dennis. In an instant, I headed out the door to see what was going on. Dennis, who obviously was not rational at the time, was in the process of "informing" the police that he did not have to pay for his groceries because he *"lived in America, and in America everyone's food is free."* As the officers started to approach Dennis, more than likely to arrest him, I interrupted the conversation and said, *"Excuse me, I'm a friend of Dennis. He has AIDS and it's starting to affect his ability to think."* As soon as I said, *"He has AIDS"* both policemen backed away from Dennis. It was apparent they had no desire to be anywhere near Dennis once learning he had AIDS.

In the early years of the AIDS epidemic, most people were afraid to touch anyone with HIV/AIDS because at that time, no one really knew how HIV could be transmitted to others. Many believed they could be infected if someone with HIV coughed, sneezed or even breathed on them. Unwittingly, I capitalized on this fear when I informed the officers of his AIDS status. Once they backed away, I helped Dennis remove the groceries from the trunk of his car, put them back in the cart and headed back to the store to pay for them. The men in blue returned to their car and drove away. As they did so, I thought, *"Who would have known that having AIDS could help prevent you from being arrested?"*

It was not only the police who were afraid of catching HIV/AIDS from Dennis. His barber, Phil, who had cut Dennis' hair for more than 10 years, considered him to be a good friend. Phil continued to cut Dennis' hair, but he'd do so only after the shop was closed. None of the other barbers working with Phil would allow Dennis in the shop once they learned he had HIV.

Dennis continued to perform his regular duties at K-State after his initial diagnosis. It was depressing for Dennis to talk to me about work once his co-workers learned of his HIV status. Almost all of his professional peers, people Dennis considered friends, started to avoid him. Even though they were trained medical professionals, they avoided Dennis because of the fear they might get infected from casual contact. In fact, many of Dennis' co-workers even refused to use the same bathroom. His department went so far as to "assign" Dennis a specific bathroom to use.

By 1987, Kansas State University officials were not comfortable having Dennis, an HIV-positive individual, as a member of the faculty. Against his wishes, Dennis was forced to "medically retire" from his position. At the time, there was quite a bit of media attention when Dennis accused K-State officials of discrimination after he was forced to retire.

One day, Dennis came into my store. I owned a gourmet-gift shop called *Kitchens Plus*. The store was also home to a restaurant, *The Croissant Café.* My café served brunch, lunch and afternoon desserts and coffee to several hundred people a day. When Dennis arrived at the store, he took a seat at the café counter and ordered a cup of coffee. While drinking his coffee, Dennis turned to the stranger sitting beside him and blurted out in a loud, cheerful voice, *"Hi, my name is Dennis. I have AIDS."*

The woman sitting beside Dennis got up immediately and left the café, as did the other three people sitting at the counter. Those sitting at the tables in the restaurant close enough to hear Dennis also left. As they did, word about Dennis having AIDS spread throughout the café. Within a matter of minutes, the café was empty. More than 50 diners left, most without finishing their lunch, and some without paying their bills. From that day on, anytime Dennis set foot in the door of *Kitchens Plus*, a member of my staff or I would immediately escort him to my office where he was out of sight, and earshot, of all the customers.

Watching my best friend deteriorate mentally was heartbreaking. I remember wondering, *"Why can't Dennis just get sick and die?"* It would have been much easier to watch Dennis deteriorate physically while still acting and thinking like the person I knew. Watching him as he became more childlike, and less like the intelligent friend I knew was almost more than I could bear.

Dennis lived on 10 acres a few miles outside of town. One day, I was with Dennis when he was driving on the two-lane road near his home. Suddenly, he pulled over into the left lane, stepped on the gas and started accelerating. Trying not to panic, I shouted, *"Dennis, what the h--- are you doing? You're on the wrong side of the road!"* He grinned and replied, *"I know – I have a new game I like to play. I drive as fast as I can on the wrong side of the road and watch people try to figure out how to get out of my way!"* That was the last day Dennis was allowed to drive. His other friends and I had no choice but to take away his car keys.

Not long after we took his keys, Dennis needed to see his doctor. At the time, the closest doctor treating AIDS patients was 60 miles away in Topeka, Kansas. Since Dennis was no longer driving, I volunteered to take him to the appointment and bring him home. When his exam was finished, it was time for lunch, so Dennis and I decided to stop at McDonald's. We were seated at a table in the dining area eating Big Macs when suddenly Dennis looked at me wide-eyed and declared, *"Don, I really have to go to the bathroom."* Before I could even comment, he jumped up from the table, unfastened his jeans and urinated on the floor in front of everyone in McDonald's.

It has been over 20 years since I watched in horror as my best friend dropped his pants to empty his bladder in the middle of McDonald's. Since that day, I have not stepped foot into another McDonald's, or eaten another Big Mac. Even today, every time I drive past a pair of those Golden Arches, I get a sick feeling in the pit of my stomach. I'll never forget that day; it was one of the saddest of my life.

Dennis finally began to deteriorate physically. He lost his appetite and began to lose weight. He claimed that nothing tasted good and the things he used to enjoy eating made him sick. One night, Dennis went out to dinner with his friend, Greg. Greg ordered both of them steak and lobster for dinner. Dennis loved his lobster. For the next three weeks, he demanded fresh lobster for breakfast, lunch and dinner. It was all he would eat. He delighted in going to the grocery store daily to pick a lobster out of the tank, take it home and watch it cook when dropped alive into a pot of boiling water. After eating nothing but lobster for three weeks, Dennis suddenly decided he *"hated lobster."*

Dennis continued to lose weight and finally ended up in the hospital. He was not hospitalized in Manhattan where we lived, because in the mid-1980s neither of the two hospitals in town would admit anyone with AIDS. To visit Dennis, I had to make a two-hour drive to a hospital in Kansas City. The first trip I made to see Dennis while he was hospitalized is one I'll never forget.

I arrived, tired from the drive and very nervous about seeing Dennis. He first told me he had HIV in March 1986. When I was tested six months later, I learned I also was HIV-positive. Dennis and I were in the "same boat." We both had the same virus, but I was still completely healthy. It was already difficult to deal with the fact that my best friend's mind was pretty much gone and wondering when I, too, would start to go "crazy." I wasn't sure I could handle seeing Dennis also seriously physically ill.

As I reluctantly approached the door to his room, my eyes filled with tears and my hands started to shake. The front of Dennis' door was covered with a huge yellow sign that said things like – "Warning – Avoid contact with blood or other bodily fluids" – "Do Not Enter without authorized medical personnel." It reminded me of a warning sign you'd see before entering a dangerously radioactive area.

Before I could go in, I followed instructions and put a paper suit over my clothes, a surgical cap over my hair, a mask over my nose and mouth, gloves on my hands and goggles over my eyes. The nurse who entered the room with me suggested, *"It would be best not to touch the patient."* I was overwhelmed when I first saw Dennis.

He was thin, pale and had aged dramatically. He stared as I entered the room. I'm sure he had no idea who the "creature" dressed from head to toe in a "hazard" suit happened to be. When I said, *"Hi Dennis"* he recognized my voice and smiled.

After only ten minutes, the nurse practically ordered me to leave. Once in the hall, I slowly removed my paper suit, cap, mask, gloves and goggles and as instructed, threw everything in a red container outside the entrance to the room. The container was emblazoned with the words "hazardous materials."

I left the hospital and climbed into my car. I had plans to stay with friends in Kansas City that night, but I couldn't bear the thought of socializing. It was dark, I was exhausted and I just wanted to go home. I drove 125 miles back to Manhattan fighting back tears the entire way.

When I first met Dennis, he was the picture of health. He had a muscular, trim build and weighed about 190 pounds. He reminded me of someone who might have been recently discharged from the Marines. The last week of his life, Dennis was bedridden, weighed less than 100 pounds and literally looked like an old man even though he was only in his 30s. Toward the end of his life, he could not talk, he just mumbled. The last few times I saw him, I'm not sure he knew me. In fact, I'm not even sure he was aware anyone was in his room.

Dennis died in June 1988; two years and one month after we met for lunch and I learned he had tested positive for HIV. He passed away after developing Pneumocystis carinii pneumonia (PCP), the most common cause of death for people with AIDS. His suffering was over. I was left to wonder when mine would begin.

Even though it has been more than 20 years since I watched my best friend suffer and die from complications of AIDS, I think about him daily. Seeing a McDonald's always brings a flood of memories – from the first day he told me he was infected, to the day I received my HIV diagnosis, to the various struggles we faced as he slowly exited this life. Dennis was an incredible man and the best of best friends. I'm blessed to have had him in my life.

Dennis accepted me for myself and rarely criticized my decisions or behavior, unless he thought I really screwed up and needed a good talking to. He always went out of his way to help with anything I needed. In other words, my friendship was important to him. Because of our bond during life, I firmly believe Dennis even went out of his way to help me after his death.

About a year or so after he died, I came home from work one beautiful afternoon. I had plans to go to dinner with friends that evening, but I had a little time to myself. I decided to sit outside with a glass of iced tea. I was curled up on the swing in my screened porch enjoying the weather and the subtle sounds of spring. My lawn was freshly manicured, my landscaped beds bursting with blooming red tulips.

Since being diagnosed with HIV, rarely did I ever feel relaxed, but on that afternoon I felt surprisingly at ease. Suddenly it felt as if someone was there. I looked up, glanced to my right, and there stood Dennis. He looked at me intently and appeared as healthy as the first day we met.

I distinctly remember my mouth dropped open. Dennis smiled and said, *"Don, I'm not supposed to be here. But I want you to know I'm OK. **Everything is wonderful** and I don't want you to be afraid."* Those words are etched in my memory, exactly as Dennis said them to me. I started to stammer as I tried to respond. Dennis smiled the warmest smile I can ever remember and disappeared.

At first, I was reluctant to mention to anyone that Dennis had come to pay me a "visit." After all, people would think that I was either lying, had dementia or was just completely nuts. However, I know that Dennis was there, either physically or subconsciously. Somehow he came to visit.

The first thing Dennis said to me was, *"Don, I'm not supposed to be here."* I believe he was stating the obvious. When we die, we're not allowed to return to visit our loved ones. After all, if we were allowed to do so, everyone would come back to reassure those left behind. I strongly believe Dennis broke the rules – maybe the most important one – so he could come back to give me a message. While Dennis was alive, he was always willing to go out of his way to help me with anything I needed. He thrived on helping a friend. After his death, I believe Dennis felt compelled to help me deal with the emotional struggles I faced everyday. Dennis needed me to know that he was not only OK, but that his life was *"wonderful."* Dennis needed me to know that someday my life would also be *"wonderful."*

When I talk about my life, I'm often asked if I'm afraid to die. I can honestly say that I have absolutely no fear of death. I'm terrified of the process I might go through to get there, but I'm not afraid to die. Thanks to Dennis, I know in my heart that we go to a better place after we die. The very last thing Dennis ever said to me was, *"I don't want you to be afraid."* And I'm not.

My encounter with Dennis helped me understand there is nothing more important in life than the relationships we have with the people we love. Money or material objects do not measure our success in life. The number of people who would be willing to break the rules, come back and let us know that *"everything is wonderful"* is what determines if our life was worth the journey.

Comments on Dennis' Story

"Dear Don ... What impacted me the most yesterday was Dennis' story because I will never look at McDonald's or the grocery store the same. It kills me to think of my best friend going through that kind of pain." – Tasha

"Dear Don ... One thing that seemed to impact me the most in your presentation was your personal experience with your

friend, Dennis. Thinking about all that you did for your friend and how much he changed really hit me hard as I imagined my friends suffering the same fate right before my eyes." – Allison

"Dear Don … I learned a lot from what you had to say. … This virus gradually kills you. It does not kill you quickly. It gives you the pain and misery first and then it kills you." – Tad

"Dear Don … When you talked about your best friend losing his mind, not having control of himself and having to wear diapers, it really made me realize that you don't just die. You have a great deal of suffering. It kind of scared me because suffering to me is a lot worse than death." – Louisa

"Don … I went home and told my mom about what you said about Dennis and how you had that dream in the hospital. She thought that was great. She also thinks it is a good idea to be educating kids about AIDS. She says that this is almost more important than learning about the other subjects in school and I agree." – Mike

"Dear Don … I learned a lot, but the most important thing that stands out the most was your description of the death process. I knew that it was a long, slow road to the end, but I never really realized how physically and emotionally painful it really is. Also, I wasn't aware of the way that AIDS patients are at the very end … not recognizing their family or friends. It must have hurt your heart to see your close friends in that position, and all I can say is that I'm sorry." – Emmi

"Dear Don … What impacted me the most about this presentation were the stories you told. It made it into a real life situation and easier to believe and understand. Your McDonald's story was horrible ... it would be terrible to have happen. I don't know how you dealt with that but it must have been hard … I can't even imagine! It shows really how awful AIDS is and I never realized that." – Sammy

"What impacted me the most is hearing that you had to change your best friend's diaper." – Chris

"Dear Don Carrel … I never really knew what happens when you get AIDS until you told us what your friends went through. I was really shocked when Dennis dropped his pants in the middle of Mickey D's and started peeing. I started to cry." – Justin

"Dear Don … On my way to class I was thinking 'This is just going to be another lecture about what I learned a long time ago.' Your speech turned out to be so much more. Hearing you speak opened my eyes and made me see I really do have something to fear. I couldn't see myself going through what Dennis went through. I couldn't even see myself going through what you are either." – Anthony

"Dear Don ... Another big eye-opener to me was when you discussed dementia. This was a major part of having the disease that I had never heard of. It seems almost like torture. ... You helped me to see that getting the disease, finding out about the disease, or even dying from the disease aren't even the hardest parts or the scariest parts of having the disease. It is going through all the painful stages and treatments, watching yourself deteriorate and break down, piece by piece." – Emily

Comments about HIV/AIDS and suicide:

When Dennis first told me he was infected with HIV, he said, *"There's nothing I can do about it now. So far, I feel fine. I'm going to continue to go to work every day and teach my classes and do my research. I'm not going to worry about it until I get sick and can't take care of myself. When I do get that sick ... I'm going to commit suicide."* While Dennis never did commit suicide, thousands of people of all ages have chosen death as an alternative to living life with HIV/AIDS.

"Don ... I have a story to tell you, you are probably tired of hearing stories, but here is one for you to think about. I had a good friend in a little town of Smithville, Mo. who killed himself a few months ago. His name was Brad. He was on the track team, football team, pep club president, National Honor Society and was the funniest, nicest and cutest boy that ever was. A week before homecoming he went to the doctor and he found out he was HIV positive ... Brad told two people, his girlfriend of 6 years and my best friend. His girlfriend went nuts & broke up with him. Homecoming night he blew his brains out while everyone was at the football game. The news was announced over the intercom and the game came to a halt, everyone went home in tears." – Christina

"Don ... there are a couple of things I wanted to write you about ... first ... when you read that letter about the student named Brad, well that story really got to me. I started crying because I knew Brad. He was one of my good friends. ... Second ... I think that one of my friends has the virus. She had sex with this guy who had AIDS. They never used condoms and she had a miscarriage with his baby. Now she has been with 4 other partners, all unprotected. ... She refuses to take a test or use condoms. What can I do to help her?" – Megan

"Don ... I can personally relate because my first love and best friend committed suicide 8 months after finding out that he had gotten HIV through a one night stand with an exotic dancer. I'll never understand why people take those chances." – China

"Dear Don ... My friend Mena was the type of person who was

always happy. One day she started acting weird, I mean depressed or something. I was curious, so I asked, and then she said she'd tell me later. After school she wanted me to meet her at the park. When I got there, she looked like she had been crying. She told me that she went to get tested for HIV and it came out positive. I couldn't believe it – my best friend – Why? The next day, her mother called me and told me Mena was dead. She blew her brains out." – Linda

"Don … A friend of mine that goes to Kansas City Academy contracted AIDS about a year and a half ago. He transmitted it to two other people before he learned he had it. One of those individuals is a girl I was with about four months ago. She called me two weeks ago to tell me she had AIDS. When we were together we were always careful, but I was still terribly frightened I might be sick. My HIV test came out negative and I was greatly relieved. My ex-girlfriend has attempted to take her life three times since that phone call and is presently under psychiatric care. There is nothing I can do." – Anonymous

"Dear Don … Last year I skipped school with my best friend because she was scared to go and find out the results of her HIV test alone. She told me I was the only person that she really trusted and she didn't want anyone else finding out that she might have AIDS. … My friend found out she did have AIDS. When I talk to her she is always so depressed. I pray sometimes that she doesn't go off and kill herself because she is always talking about how she hates living." – Anonymous

"Dear Don … I had a friend and his name was David. He found out that he was HIV positive … he was 13 when he found out he was infected and he died when he was 15. He slit his wrists because his family turned against him and so did everyone except me." – Laneya

"Dear Don … The stories you told our class brought tears to my eyes. They really make you think about how special life is. It made me think that life is too short to do stupid things. I feel like I've known you a long time. My friend's Dad had AIDS and shortly after he found out he took a gun and blew his brains out. My friend is still sad. Just looking at her makes me so sad. … Once you get AIDS, there's no going back in time to change your actions. … I think you are one of the coolest people I've ever met. … I bet you have saved millions of teenagers from getting AIDS. So thank-you. Thank-you. Thank you a million times. I really think you were sent from Heaven to help us teenagers." – Jennifer

"Dear Mr. Don … I would like to say thank you for coming. … Even though you had me crying. You might not remember but I'm the one who came up to you with my best friend. We were telling you about how my brother died from AIDS … well actually he committed suicide because he caught the disease *from his girlfriend and she killed herself and so did he. ... I would like to say thanks for coming and sharing your life experience with us. I give all the love and blessing to you. God bless you and keep your spirit up high." – Love Always, Ashlei*

Comments - Dennis – the ghost

Suddenly I had the strangest sensation of being watched. It felt as if someone was there. I looked up, glanced to my right and there stood Dennis. He was looking at me intently and appeared as healthy as he did the first day we met.

I distinctly remember my mouth dropped open. Dennis smiled and said, *"Don, I'm **not** supposed to be here. But I want you to know I'm OK. **Everything is wonderful** and I don't want you to be afraid."*

"Dear Don ... I'm sorry that you had to see your best friend die because of this virus. I believe that he is in heaven watching over you. J" – Katie

"Dear Don ... Your story about seeing Dennis after his death was great. I think you were telling the truth and I know it could happen. He must have been a great friend. You had to have been a true friend to have not abandoned him." – Jeremy

"Dear Don ... My favorite part about you speaking was the story of your friend coming back after he had died. I had an encounter like that after my Grandpa died and nobody believed me about it. But I know I saw him." – Serena

"Dear Don ... I'm sorry about your friend Dennis ... I know people have already told you that they believed your ghost story about Dennis, but I have seen the ghost of my dog, so I have to believed it. ... Don, you had my attention the whole time ... I might have laughed when you said Dennis pissed all over in McDonald's, but it was out of astonishment." – Austin

"Dear Don ... It is very neat to know that your friend came back and told you he was okay and safe in heaven. Our family had a similar experience like that. My great-grandpa was still alive, but very sick, and he saw angels. Now, I know that everything will be okay once I die. ... Thanks for coming and sharing your stories." – Kimberly

"Dear Don ... I loved all of your stories. My favorite story was about your friend who came back to you as a ghost. I think your dream about living so you can come back and talk to people about AIDS is definitely some sort of sign. What you're

*doing with your life is neat. ... I know that I will never get AIDS.
I have chosen to never have sex until I am married. And my
husband will be tested. I have never, and will never take drugs
either. I know I am safe." – Anonymous*

Comments about AIDS phobia:

It wasn't just the police who were afraid of catching HIV/AIDS
from Dennis.

*"Dear Mr. Don ... people can still be very cruel. I have this
friend who told me the other day she would never touch or
stand by a person who has AIDS. It really hurt me to hear her
say that and in a way made me mad. I told her she couldn't get
AIDS just by touching or standing by someone. She said her
mother brought her up that way and still she wouldn't go or
touch them. My parents feel a little uncomfortable with me
touching a person who has AIDS, but I don't care what they
think or feel because I don't have a problem with anyone who
has AIDS or any other disease. To me that's how everyone
should be. I think if I got AIDS I would want to die right then
because I wouldn't want to go through the things your friends
and you have to go through. ... To stand up and tell your story
takes a lot of courage." – Nicole*

*" Dear Don ... I must admit before you came, I was a little afraid
of being around people with AIDS. Now I know you can only get
AIDS from sex or sharing needles. I have never had sex or
shared a needle before, but now thanks to you I will think twice
before I have sex. ... The life situation you are in and the stories that you shared are really influencing and I believe it can
happen. You are a great person and you have made a big
impact on lots of kid's lives." – Staci*

*"Dear Don ... Not only did you teach me about how AIDS can
be transmitted through sex, you also did an excellent job of
clearing up some of the phobias some of us feel about AIDS
victims. I know that I can never get AIDS by touching or hugging someone with the disease, but you showed me how to be
more comfortable around these people. After your speech all
of us talked in the hall about how scared we are to have sex
now. That will let you know you are reaching people and
changing lives." – Phil*

*"Dear Don ... My family has endured the loss of a loved one to
AIDS also. However, my uncle, the man that died from AIDS,
acquired the disease during the 80s. I don't know the exact
year because my parents, both in the medical profession, iso-
lated him from our family in fear of our health. It wasn't until 2*

months prior to his death that I found out he was dying of AIDS. Your stories helped me to understand my family's actions; not to say they did the right thing, simply to understand." – Carolyn

CHAPTER 5

My "Kid Brother" – Kenny

I met Kenny in the summer of 1987. He had recently moved to Manhattan, Kansas, and had stumbled upon my café. After seeing him come in a number of times one week, I introduced myself. He quickly became a regular customer, stopping into *The Croissant Café* six or seven days a week, and sometimes even twice on the same day. His typical schedule included eating lunch and then hanging around for three or four hours drinking coffee.

One afternoon, I joined him at his table to get to know my newest "regular." Kenny was not very tall, on the slender side, had dark curly hair and a cute baby face. Had it not been for his short, slightly scruffy beard and mustache, he would have easily passed for a high school student. Given his unhurried schedule and his appearance, I assumed he was taking classes at Kansas State University. Believing he was a college student, I started the conversation by asking him about the classes he was taking at K-State. He shook his head and replied, *"I don't go to K-State – I'm not in college."* Intrigued, I asked what type of job he had that allowed him to spend almost every afternoon in my café. Kenny, who was 23 at the time, answered, *"I don't have a job – I'm retired."*

Seeing my shocked expression, Kenny launched into his personal story. I think he had been waiting for me to ask him about his life, and I was amazed at his ability to share the details that he revealed that afternoon. It began simply enough. As a child, Kenny dreamed of growing up and joining the Air Force, like his dad. When Kenny graduated from high school at age 19, he enlisted in the Air Force.

Within two years after enlisting, Kenny's health started to deteriorate. In a matter of a few months, he had hepatitis, constant colds, fevers and numerous skin sores. In January 1985, Kenny was hospitalized for tests to determine why he was continuously ill. The results of his tests were far worse than anything Kenny, his doctors or his parents had ever imagined. The day before Kenny's 21st birthday, he received an unbelievable diagnosis: he had full-blown AIDS. On more than one occasion, Kenny said to me, *"Most people get something special for their 21st birthday. Not me; all I remember getting was AIDS."*

According to Kenny, the Air Force kicked him out a few months later. If you are in the military today and find out you have HIV/AIDS, you are not discharged. But in the mid-1980s, when not much was understood about HIV and the ways it could be transmitted to others, the military automatically discharged anyone infected with the virus.

For the first year following his unceremonious discharge, Kenny did not receive any disability pay from the Air Force. HIV/AIDS was a new disease, and the branches of the military did not have a disability policy in place for it. Finally, after a year of intense physical and financial struggle, Kenny started receiving a monthly disability check of $1,100. As often happens with payments given for a disability, he was told he would continue to receive $1,100 every month until he died, unless he went back to work, in which case, his checks would be discontinued.

With no incentive to find a job, it is no wonder Kenny found refuge in my café. It was the one place where he could fit in and find a purpose, even if that purpose was just to chat with other customers.

Kenny moved to Kansas so that he could be closer to his parents who had retired in the area. At the time, $1,100 a month was just enough money for him to rent a small apartment, put gas in his beloved Volkswagen and come into my café to have lunch. Kenny appeared to be in fairly good health when I met him, but he had no reason or desire to look for a job. He was afraid to give up his disability and go to work. He knew if he did so, and then got sick again and wasn't able to work, he would have no paycheck and no disability check.

Kenny frequently mentioned that he felt worthless because he didn't have a career. He believed he had nothing to contribute to society. Kenny felt as if his life had no purpose.

This sense of worthlessness went beyond his career aspirations. In the two years I knew Kenny, he rarely had a date. If he did go out with anyone, the relationship ended soon after his HIV-positive status was disclosed. In the 1980s, no one wanted to date anyone with HIV. Almost no one would even touch someone with HIV and would never consider drinking out of the same glass as someone who was infected. The idea of kissing or having sex with someone with AIDS was terrifying, even with proper protection.

In fact, it was unprotected sex earlier in his life that brought Kenny to this point. He believed he had become infected with HIV the first time he had sex. How old was Kenny when he first had sex? I remember him telling me he was only 14. Kenny's mom, Christel, remembers him telling her he was 16 at the time. In either case, Kenny was convinced his infection occurred the first time he made the decision to become sexually active.

Kenny was only 23 when we first met, and I was 36. I was an adult trying to cope with having HIV. However, unlike Kenny, I had already been blessed with a family and a successful business, and had experienced some of the advantages everyone hopes to have when he or she becomes an adult. In my mind, Kenny was "just a kid." He was a young man who never had a chance to do many of the things everyone takes for granted once they reach adulthood.

When I share Kenny's story, what I try to illustrate is that long before HIV/AIDS affects anyone physically, it starts to take away the dreams, hopes and expectations you have for your life; things you take for granted. Having AIDS destroyed Kenny's life-long dream of being in the Air Force. It destroyed Kenny's career. Having AIDS prevented Kenny from the likelihood of enjoying a serious, loving relationship with another person. If you have HIV/AIDS it will, without doubt, reduce or eliminate the possibility of marriage or having a family.

I had a great deal of respect and admiration for Kenny. During the brief time I knew him, I rarely heard him complain about his situation, and he always had a smile on his face. Kenny had an incredible smile, one that was accompanied by bright and twinkling eyes. When he smiled at anyone, even strangers, he almost always received a smile in return. During our friendship, Kenny spent hundreds of hours at the counter in *The Croissant Café* drinking coffee and carrying on conversations with anyone who would listen.

I will never forget the day Kenny died. It was October 22, 1988. Kenny was in the hospital that day, and I had promised him I would visit about noon so we could have lunch together. It was cold outside, far colder than it had been any day since the previous winter. *Kitchens Plus* was packed with shoppers that morning. The weather had brought in a lot of people who suddenly seemed to realize it was the end of October and they'd not even started their holiday shopping. In addition, *The Croissant Café* was packed, and a long line of people stood waiting for tables. My café was one of the few places in Manhattan serving homemade soups, and since it was bitterly cold, it seemed as if everyone in town wanted hot soup for lunch.

When it was time for me to leave for the hospital to meet Kenny for lunch, I looked around my store and café. Both were swamped. I decided we were just too busy for me to leave. I would go visit Kenny later, once the rush was over.

I arrived at the hospital about 3:00 p.m. I hurried down the hall and pushed open the door to Kenny's room – but he wasn't there. The bed in the room had been stripped of sheets, and the mattress was bare. I was still holding the door open when I noticed one of the nurses hurrying down the hall toward me. As she approached, I asked, *"Where's Kenny?"* The nurse walked up to me, put her arm on my shoulder and replied, *"I'm so sorry, Don, but Kenny passed away about 15 minutes ago."*

Fifteen minutes. I missed the death of someone I had grown to love as a kid brother because I chose my business over my friend. I had no idea Kenny was going to die that day. I thought we had more time. I thought Kenny had more time. He had been hospitalized many times in the previous six months, but he would always recover enough to go home for a week or two before he would relapse and end up back in the hospital. I had expected this time would be no different, but I was wrong.

I have no idea how long I stood in the doorway of his hospital room processing what just happened. Even today, more than 20 years after Kenny's death, **I have never forgiven myself for being three hours late to lunch.**

When Kenny died at 2:45 p.m. that day, he was only 24 years old. He weighed 67 pounds. He was wearing diapers. But he did not die alone. His mother, Christel, and his father, Richard, were at his bedside. Kenny's mother, held him in her arms as he took his last breath. According to her, *"It was not an easy death. Kenny died of respiratory failure, which means he drowned in his own mucous. How I wish I could have traded places."*

Before his death, Kenny battled a number of horrific diseases heroically. These included PCP; Mycobacterium avium complex (MAC), a severe infection that enters through the lungs or intestines and spreads through the bloodstream causing fever, night sweats, weight loss, pain and diarrhea; and Kaposi's sarcoma, an AIDS-related cancer. To add insult to injury, in the last few weeks of his life, like my friend Dennis, Kenny's mind had started to deteriorate from AIDS-related dementia. Even though Kenny lived in Manhattan, Kansas, his parents often had to drive him 125 miles to Kansas City, Missouri, when he needed to be hospitalized. When Kenny first moved to town none of the local hospitals would admit AIDS patients.

I received an email from Kenny's mom after his death. Christel knew I talked to others about Kenny, and I shared with her on a number of occasions what an incredible impact his story had on everyone who heard it. She was proud that Kenny, even after his death, was helping teach others how to protect themselves from HIV/AIDS. Christel closed her email by writing, *"We are thinking of you often. You are a very special person and it seems you have a mission, let's hope you will be able to reach many young people, because what Kenny went through, no one should ever have to. We are impressed by your drive and your goals are the best, stay on it. We love you always, Richard and Christel."*

The Impact of Kenny's Story

The impact that Kenny is having on those who hear his story is amazing. Of all the "stories" I share with people, the one about Kenny is the one I receive the most comments about. I have told others about Kenny thousands of times, yet I still easily tear up when sharing my memories of him. Those hearing his story are also often brought to tears.

"Don ...What impacted me the most about your lesson was just that man Kenny. How you said, he would come and drink coffee just waiting for his life to end. That made me think about

how sad and bad AIDS is. It's so easy to not get AIDS I don't want any of my friends to get it. You <u>really</u> impacted my life and I will never forget you." – Jennifer

"Don ... What opened my eyes was when you explained how lonely AIDS really is, and how it destroys all your hopes and aspirations." – Carl

"Don ... I learned so much from you. I just kept picturing my best friend in a diaper and I kept thinking, why should anyone have to go through that? I am so sorry that you did. ... I cried, for me, for you, and for all the people I know and love." – Andrea

"Don ... I have been learning about AIDS since seventh grade. ... They don't tell us how AIDS patients die. I think they keep that from us because they think we are too fragile to hear it. Your explanation was terrifying. It makes you think about a lot of things." – Danielle

"Don ... I knew what AIDS was, how it was contracted, and that you eventually die from it; but I had no idea what it was like to have the virus. If schools would go more into detail on the effects of AIDS, I think more people would listen and finally begin to grasp the true danger of it." – Cara

"Dear Don ... After you talked about your friend Kenny it made me think about how he used to be just like me and then went on to have to wear a diaper. It scared me to think about how a close friend could have that happen to them. The most important thing I learned was to always use protection, because anyone could have AIDS. I will always remember what happened to Kenny." – Conor

"Dear Mr. Carrel ... The story that impacted me the most was about your friend, Kenny. It really made me realize that HIV could affect the way you live for the rest of your life and could ruin any dreams you have for your future. I now know that I want to do everything in my power to prevent myself from getting HIV. After hearing your story, I feel so lucky. It is easy for me to say that I don't have HIV now ... but for you, it must be difficult to realize that you already have HIV and there is nothing you can do to get rid of it. ... You have persevered and used this as an opportunity to educate other people to make sure they don't have to live the life that you have to endure. I respect you greatly for that." – Nicole

"Dear Don ... I'm so sorry for what has happened to you and Kenny and I learned so much that it's not even a question as to if I will abstain till marriage ... You seem like a really cool guy, you seem really nice, it makes me realize that it can happen to anyone. ... I'm pretty sure you saved someone's life today." – Jacob

"Dear Don … The story about your friend Kenny was really touching. That he could get infected the very first time he had sex is a very powerful message. It shows how anyone can get AIDS." – Nora

"Dear Don … I didn't realize the disease could take everything away from you. I thought you could just live normally and then die." – Adam

"Dear Don … Your stories helped me understand that anyone can get AIDS and that no matter what your dreams and ambitions are, AIDS can take all of them away." – Jake

Dear Don … Your presentations really changed the way I think about stuff now. I used to think that getting HIV at my age could never happen. But after you told us about your friend, Kenny, who got it the first time he had sex, it made me stop and think about my actions." – Cody

"Dear Don … You showed me that I don't want to get this virus. … I couldn't go through life not being able to find someone to love and start a family with. I couldn't do it. I want a family. I want to spend my life with someone in a very intimate relationship. I knew I was going to wait before having sex and you talking gave me more reasons why I shouldn't have sex." – Anonymous

"Dear Mr. Carrel …AIDS is very serious and it's really cool of you for coming and talking to us. Last year my 14-year-old friend got AIDS. She tried to sleep around after that but too many people found out about it. … I'm waiting until I get married to have any kind of sex." – Missy

"Dear Don … First of all, I want to tell you how sorry I am about your friends. I know what it's like to be alone without your best friend and it's really hard. I bet it was even harder for you to watch your friends pass away and think that there was nothing you could do for them but you're wrong. You did a lot by being there for them, making them smile, or laugh and just sitting next to them in complete silence. You'll always treasure those memories and so will they. That's what best friends are all about." – Amanda

"Dear Don … I'm ashamed to admit that when I heard we would have a guest speaker I was less than thrilled. I thought to myself, "Here we go again, some boring person to throw some boring statistics at us and preach to us about how we should all be chaste angels who never do anything bad ever." Then you started to talk. You were different than the other speakers we've had. You didn't just talk at us, but you talked to us. … You told us your life stories and presented what you had in a way that we could relate to. … You presented yourself as a person. … I was particularly affected by the story of your friend

Kenny. I'm sorry for your loss and I know he is in a better place now, applauding you and your efforts." – Chaise

"Dear Don ... On a personal note I have lost a close friend to AIDS. It gave me chills when you described the deterioration of your friend's health. ... I just want you to know that some of us <u>were</u> listening. ... I will never use needles. I am also a virgin at 18 and am in no hurry to change that. Be aware of what you've done ... you've made a friend forever, <u>not</u> <u>for</u> <u>life</u>, forever." – Justin

"Dear Don ... Thank you for talking to us about AIDS and the lifetime effects it has on people. Your discussion was touching, heartfelt and most of all, extremely educational. Never has anyone impacted me in such a dramatic influential way. ... You taught me that it's not death it's the suffering that one should be afraid of. You are truly God sent." – Vera

"Dear Don ... Wow, where do I begin? ... You left us pondering what it would be like to have AIDS, but it's something we want to ponder, not experience. The dreams we've tried to fulfill ... could all vanish within one night of what we thought at the time happened to be "fun." ... I have learned a lot from your speech and I think that it is a very good message you send to young people. ... I would like all my friends and even enemies, to hear this. ... You have forever impacted me and hopefully other students." – Keri

"Dear Don ... All throughout school, we are always given statistics & are told what we should and shouldn't do. Your presentation really helped me & many other students to see HIV and AIDS affecting real people. The stories you shared about your two friends who died was the part of your presentation that I know will stay with me for a long time, if not forever. ... Listening to you speak today, inspired me to do all I can to help those people in need." – Lauren

"Dear Don ... To get back to your personal stories, this was an extremely eye-opening situation! When you asked us to picture ourselves changing our best friend's diaper, it almost made me cry. This made me make the decision to stay away from sexual activities (for as long as possible) and the use of IV drugs. ... To end this letter, your presentation touched my life. I will always remember the advice you gave our class." – Meredith

CHAPTER 6

"I'm interrupting
this presentation to ..."

So far, you have "heard" – or should I say – you have read, the first two parts of my "presentation." I shared information about myself and told you about Dennis and Kenny, two of my friends who lost their lives to AIDS.

Normally, I would take an "emotional break" and discuss the history of HIV and some of the statistics associated with the disease. If you'd prefer to continue with my "presentation," skip ahead to the chapter titled the "History of HIV." If you're interested in learning in depth about my personal struggle with HIV and AIDS, keep reading.

I normally share little about how my life has changed since learning I have HIV. I'm frequently asked why I don't talk more about how I personally deal with having AIDS or how my family and friends reacted to my illness. One reason is that I prefer to describe what it's like living with HIV/AIDS through stories about my friends, especially Kenny. Most of my audiences consist of teenagers and young adults, and I have always believed that younger age groups would connect to Kenny's story more than my own. After all, Kenny was infected with HIV when he was a teenager.

This reason, while true, is not the primary reason I talk more about my friends who battled HIV/AIDS and not much about myself. To be honest, it's just too painful for me to share a lot of details about my personal struggle. During the first 20 years of my diagnosis, it took everything I had to survive emotionally. At one point, I nearly became an alcoholic, and I seriously considered suicide on more than one occasion. Whenever I talk in detail about my life with HIV/AIDS, I feel as if I'm reliving the experience. Living through those years once was enough.

I'm not sure it's even possible to explain how I've been able to handle the emotional and physical rollercoaster since the first day I suspected I might have HIV. I'm convinced I was in shock for most of the first five years I knew about my infection. I vividly remember some events that occurred during the early years of my infection, but have almost no memory of what was happening in my everyday life.

In this chapter, and several that follow, I will reveal how having HIV has impacted my life in more detail than I've ever done previously. I'll also share thoughts from family, friends and loved ones to help answer the questions I often get about their reaction to discovering they had a son, brother, father or friend with AIDS.

Life before my HIV test

Before I expand my story, there is something I need to share. I'm gay. During the early years of HIV/AIDS, most Americans were under the impression that only gay or bisexual men could be infected with HIV. In fact, AIDS was considered to be a "gay disease."

In the earliest days of the AIDS epidemic, most Americans, even those studying the virus at the Centers for Disease Control (CDC), thought HIV only infected men who had sex with men (MSM). It was in 1980 when the first four Americans died from complications of AIDS. All four happened to be gay men. In 1981 and early 1982, it appeared that primarily gay men were getting infected. In fact, the CDC first nicknamed this new disease GRID: gay-related immune deficiency.

However, throughout the rest of the world, HIV/AIDS was spreading in the general population without regard to sexual orientation. Worldwide 85 percent of those with HIV/AIDS were heterosexual, and only 15 percent of infected individuals were homosexual. Global statistics clearly illustrated that AIDS was not a gay disease.

While it was true that during the early 1980s nearly all the Americans who contracted HIV were MSM, the same is not true today. Currently in the United States, nearly half of new HIV infections occur in those who are heterosexual – especially women, teenagers and people of color. Later in this book, in the chapter titled "Patient Zero," I'll explain the most widely accepted theory as to why those infected with HIV early in this country were primarily gay or bisexual men.

While I'm gay and have AIDS, being gay has nothing to do with contracting HIV. Nearly 100 percent of those who contract HIV do so because they have unprotected sex with someone infected with the virus, or they share a needle during IV drug use with someone infected with the virus. HIV does not discriminate; all it needs is a suitable host.

If asked about my sexual orientation during a presentation, I'm always honest with my answer. However, there are two reasons I don't normally reveal this personal aspect about myself unless asked. The primary reason is simply because anyone who partici-pates in risky sexual behavior is at risk of HIV/AIDS, regardless of gender or sexual orientation. The second reason is that revealing the fact I'm gay, while not an issue for most of those in my audience, is sometimes an issue for the parents of those who hear me speak. On a few occasions, I've been accused of "promoting my gay agenda" by people who have not seen or heard my presentation. No one who has actually heard me speak has ever made this accu-sation.

My one and only objective when sharing my story is for those lis-tening to learn what they need to know to make safer decisions about drug use and sexual behavior. Every time I have the privilege to speak to any group, I say a silent prayer asking that no one in the room ever contracts HIV. To help accomplish this goal, it is vital that those listening believe I'm truthful. If the subject comes up, reveal-ing the fact I'm gay adds to my credibility.

I wasn't aware of my sexual orientation early in my adult life. When I was growing up, there were no gay or lesbian characters on television, there were no positive gay/lesbian role models and the topic was almost never discussed. What I do remember hearing were negative stereotypical descriptions that were and are not true. For example, all gay men *"wear makeup and dresses"* and all les-bians *"wear flannel shirts, drive pick-ups and hate men."* I was told that homosexuals were focused only on sex and had no interest in long-term relationships or in having a "family."

While growing up, I learned it was "normal" as an adult to get married, have children and live with your family in a nice house somewhere in the suburbs. I had an extremely strong desire, start-ing in early childhood, to grow up and have the perfect relationship and family. As far as I knew at the time, getting married was the first step in achieving this dream.

During college, I met Karen, my future wife. Karen and I dated for three years while we finished our degrees at K-State. We had a lot of fun doing all the crazy things college students do and made many friends. I proposed to her during our last year of college, and we were married three months after graduation. Our oldest son, Christopher, was born two years later and our second son, Matthew, two and a half years after that.

Five years into our marriage, I had achieved my childhood dreams. I had a wife and two beautiful children. Even though I was only in my 20s, I already had been very successful in the insurance and investment business. Karen and I lived in a beautiful home in one of the nicest neighborhoods in town. We also had acquired three pieces of investment property. Our family and friends thought we had the perfect life.

However, something wasn't quite right. Karen and I had a lot of fun together and enjoyed socializing with other couples in situations similar to our own. We never argued. Karen was my best friend, and I loved her. Despite my wishing otherwise, my true sexual orientation started to emerge and in a matter of a few months, I knew I was gay. One evening, I shamefully told Karen. Being the loving wife and friend she was, Karen gracefully accepted the situation, and we agreed to divorce. Ending our marriage was extremely difficult for both of us.

When our divorce was final, my sons were young. Chris had just turned four and Matt was only 18 months old. At the time, I felt like a complete failure. My lifetime goal of having the perfect loving family had come to an abrupt end, and I rightfully blamed myself.

To say I was depressed is an understatement. I lost complete interest in my career. My profession required me to spend my time making recommendations to others about how to protect their families financially. I couldn't handle talking to others about taking care of their families when I had just completely destroyed my own.

The next year was brutal. Like most married couples, the friends Karen and I made were primarily other married couples. It was the late 1970s and people, in general, were not as comfortable having gay friends as they are today. Most of my friends, especially the men, would have nothing to do with me once they discovered I was gay. I was tossed aside by nearly all of my so-called friends. The occasional cocktail or beer I had previously enjoyed having with them turned into more and more frequent drinking – most of it done while alone at home.

Eventually, I started to meet a few other men and women who were gay and lesbian and began to make new friends. I also started dating a few people and began having sex again. When I first began dating after my divorce, AIDS was unheard of. It was quite common to date someone for a short time and end up in bed. Condoms were never used.

Over the next few years I dated a number of people, including a man named Jim who lived three hours away in Omaha, Nebraska. Jim and I dated for about three or four months and parted ways because neither of us cared to continue a long-distance relationship or relocate to another city.

In 1983, I met Scott, another formerly married man who also had made the decision to get a divorce because he was gay. Scott had children, something we had in common, and after dating for about six months, we moved in together.

Before Scott and I met, I don't remember hearing much about the "new" disease that was killing people in New York, Los Angeles and San Francisco. There was little information in the mainstream press. The gay community first started to learn a few details about the disease through word of mouth from friends and acquaintances or from articles starting to appear in publications, commonly called "bar rags," which were passed out in bars and restaurants that catered primarily to gay and bisexual men.

I do not recall seeing anything about the disease in the newspaper or on TV until about 1983 or 1984 and even then, there was little indication the disease was anything for the average person to worry about contracting.

By 1985, information about HIV/AIDS included more details and the news became more alarming. The number of those infected with HIV and dying of AIDS was skyrocketing. This disease was now a full-blown epidemic. I followed the information about AIDS in the news, but was not very concerned. At the time, I didn't know anyone with HIV/AIDS, plus I had been in a monogamous relationship for the last few years. There was no way I could possibly be infected with HIV, or so I thought.

On a beautiful summer afternoon in 1985, I came home from work and decided to grab something to drink and sit outside to read the paper. I lived in a small bungalow built in 1915 that I had purchased from the original owners. They had done little to upgrade it over the years, so I spent many hours remodeling and modernizing the inside of my home, but never made any changes that would affect the house's quaint exterior. Across the entire front of the house was a screened porch with the original porch swing. Over the years, I spent hundreds of hours on my porch swing, and it was there I settled in to relax and read the paper.

To my surprise, the paper that day contained a half page article about HIV and AIDS. It was the longest and most detailed article on the subject I had ever seen. The article talked about the different ways someone could get infected with HIV, and explained how once you were infected the virus attacked the immune system. After HIV had damaged the immune system significantly, an infected person would begin to suffer from multiple illnesses and eventually develop full-blown AIDS. The article went so far as to describe some of the early symptoms of the disease. Some common symptoms of those with advanced HIV included one or more of the following: swollen lymph glands, a low-grade fever that rarely goes away, shingles (a painful rash caused by the chicken pox virus), thrush (a "slimy" mouth fungus) and night sweats.

Night sweats occur while you are sleeping. You feel perfectly fine when you go to bed, but in the middle of the night you sweat profusely. It's similar to what might happen when you have a high fever and wake up with damp sheets after your fever breaks. However, night sweats are much more obvious. When you awake, your clothes are soaked, your sheets and blankets are soaked, and the mattress is soaked. It's almost as if someone emptied a bucket of water on you while you were sleeping.

After reading about night sweats being a possible symptom of HIV infection, I literally broke out in a cold sweat. I distinctly remembered that Jim, the man I dated briefly before meeting Scott, sweat profusely while he was sleeping. In the morning the sheets and blankets would be soaked. I didn't think much about it at the time. But after reading this newspaper article, it suddenly occurred to me, **I had sex four years earlier with someone who had night sweats – someone who might actually have had AIDS.**

When Scott and I began our relationship, no one really knew enough about HIV to worry about contracting it. When I realized I might have contracted the virus from Jim, or possibly someone else I had been involved with before Scott, I was instantly terrified. **It dawned on me that I actually might be infected with HIV.**

I wanted to deny there was any possibility I might be infected. After all, I wasn't sick and I had not been sick in years. I had never had night sweats. I assured myself there was nothing to worry about, but in the back of my mind, I wondered.

During the next year, the news about HIV/AIDS became even more depressing. The number of those dying was multiplying rapidly. It was becoming apparent that AIDS had a fatality rate approaching 100 percent. I continued to remain healthy and did not have a single symptom of the disease. As the months passed, the fear I felt about possibly having HIV diminished, and I found myself worrying less.

Then in March 1986, when Dennis and I had lunch, everything changed. Out of the blue, I learned my best friend was infected with HIV. Up to that point, I didn't know anyone with the disease. If my closest friend had somehow managed to get infected, couldn't the same thing have just as easily happened to me?

From that day on, I worried constantly about when Dennis would start to get sick and how soon he would die. On that day, I also took another step toward accepting the fact I might have HIV. Instead of believing I couldn't possibly have HIV, I started to believe that it was possible I might have the same fatal disease as Dennis.

One evening in the summer of 1986, about a year after I sat on my porch and read the newspaper article about night sweats, my phone rang. The man calling asked to speak to "Don Carrel." The caller identified himself as a friend of Jim, the same Jim I had been involved with years earlier. The man on the phone was calling everyone in Jim's address book to notify them that, *"Jim has AIDS and is in a hospital in Phoenix. I suggest you give him a call as soon as possible if you'd like to talk to him before he dies."* As I listened to the caller, I became light-headed and felt as if I was about to be sick to my stomach. My hands started shaking as I gripped the phone and continued the conversation. My worst fear had just been confirmed. A person I dated years earlier, someone I had been sexually involved with, now had AIDS. Before I finished the call, my eyes filled with tears. Once I hung up, I started to cry.

I don't remember much of what happened during the next couple of weeks. I tried to convince myself that everything was all right. I looked completely healthy and felt great. It had been years since I had been sick. I was trying to hang on to a shred of hope that I did **not** have HIV. However, I was afraid. The fear I felt knowing I had actually had sex with someone who was now dying of AIDS was gut-wrenching.

It was a couple of weeks before I built up enough nerve to tell Scott about the phone call. Scott was not only scared, he was furious. We had been together in a monogamous relationship for three years before I received that fateful phone call. During our years together we'd never practiced safer sex. We'd never used condoms. Suddenly, it was abundantly clear that if either one of us had HIV at the beginning of our relationship; it was likely both of us were now infected.

HIV testing was available as early as 1985, but initially, the test was rarely recommended for several reasons. One reason was that at the time, there was no treatment available for anyone with HIV/AIDS. With no medication to fight the disease, testing was not encouraged, even for those who suspected they might have the virus. Those in the same situation as the one Scott and I found ourselves in were simply told to either abstain from sex or to have safer sex to minimize the chance of spreading the infection to anyone else.

Another reason HIV testing was initially discouraged was because of the stigma attached to anyone who had HIV/AIDS. Early in the epidemic, people were terrified to be around anyone with the disease. Fear of those with AIDS was due to the uncertainty about how the virus could and could not be passed from person to person. At the time, many people were under the impression you could contract HIV simply from being in the same room with someone who was infected, especially if the person coughed or sneezed. In general, people feared touching anyone infected with HIV.

After much discussion, Scott and I decided that we weren't going to be tested for HIV at that time. We both felt fine. We also knew there was no medication currently available for treatment even if we were infected. Since our relationship was exclusive, if we were HIV-positive, there was no possibility we could infect anyone else. We agreed to try and not worry about it and to wait to get tested when medical treatment became available. However, just because we agreed to not worry didn't mean we could avoid doing so. We agonized over it constantly.

My HIV test

One day in September of 1986, Scott decided to have an HIV test without my knowledge. Since we had no symptoms, Scott was convinced his test would confirm he didn't have HIV. Scott envisioned coming home to tell me the good news, that he was not infected and then I would be tested and receive the same good news. He assumed that once we learned that neither of us had HIV, the stress we were living under would end.

When I came home from work the day Scott received his test results, I found him tearful and angry. Through the tears, Scott blurted, *"I have HIV and it's your fault."* Not long afterwards, our relationship ended.

I felt awful. More than likely, Scott was right. I probably infected him with HIV. After all, I had been involved with Jim, who subsequently died from AIDS. I didn't know Jim had HIV. I had not knowingly infected Scott. But just the same, the circumstances led me to believe I had transmitted the virus to someone I loved.

Once Scott learned he was HIV-positive, I decided to get tested. I needed to know if I was infected. Part of me still clung to a shred of hope I didn't have the disease. After all, it was possible that Scott had contracted HIV before we met, and I had somehow managed to avoid becoming infected.

There were few doctors doing HIV testing at that time and to my knowledge not a single one in town offered testing or treatment for the disease. The closest doctor screening for HIV was Dr. William Wade in Topeka, Kansas. Topeka was 60 miles from home. At the time I lived in Manhattan, Kansas, a college town about 120 miles west of Kansas City and the home of Kansas State University. Topeka was halfway between Manhattan and Kansas City, where I grew up.

The first time I saw Dr. Wade, I drove an hour just to have one tube of blood drawn and was told to come back in two weeks for the test results. The next two weeks were the longest of my life.

Two weeks later, more scared than I had ever been in my life, I made the hour trip to Topeka. I dreaded picking up my test results – I expected the news was going to be horrible, but I prayed that I was wrong. Dr. Wade didn't beat around the bush. The first thing he said was, *"Don, I'm sorry, but you do have HIV, the virus that causes AIDS ... I suggest you get your affairs in order. Based on what we know about this disease, you will be sick within a year and more than likely you will die within two."*

I left the doctor's office immediately. **I definitely had HIV.** There was no longer a reason to pray it was not true. Almost in a trance, I climbed into my car to begin the 60-mile drive home. Within minutes, I had the gas pedal to the floor, and my Honda Prelude was racing down Interstate 70 at well over 100 miles per hour. My initial instinct was to drive off the road and kill myself. I watched the right side of the interstate and looked for the best place to head for the ditch to increase the chance my accident would be fatal.

Suddenly, I burst into tears. How could I commit suicide? I had two children. Chris was 11, and my youngest, Matt, was only eight. I loved my sons and desperately wanted to watch them grow up. I did not want to be remembered as the father who had killed himself.

I took my foot off the accelerator, pulled onto the shoulder of the road and stopped the car. I put my head on the steering wheel and sobbed. If I committed suicide, I would never see my sons again. But if I didn't kill myself, I would likely die within two years. Which death would be the easiest for Chris and Matt to bear? I felt hopeless.

I began to pray. *"Dear God, I don't care what happens to me, but please don't let me die until Matt gets out of high school."* The doctor had just given me two years to live; I had just asked God for 10.

Obviously, Dr. Wade was incorrect. It has been 25 years since I was tested for HIV, and I'm still alive and well. However, I had four other friends who were diagnosed with HIV the same year I was tested. All four of them were given the same two-year notice from their doctor. During the next few years, I watched in horror as they each deteriorated physically and mentally as HIV destroyed their immune systems. They continued their decline and within two years they had all developed full-blown AIDS. By the end of three years, all four were dead.

I, on the other hand, remained completely healthy. Or maybe I should say I was physically healthy. Emotionally, I was terrified.

Every time I woke up with a runny nose, a slight fever, an upset stomach or even a bruise, I thought it was the beginning of the end. Whenever anyone I knew with HIV had a new physical problem crop up, it was a reminder my time was coming. I lived every day feeling as if I was walking around with an "ax" over my head. I wondered constantly when it was going to fall.

The birth of *Kitchens Plus*

When I was tested for HIV in 1986, I owned a retail store and restaurant. My store, *Kitchens Plus*, was similar to a Crate and Barrel. I carried all types of things for the kitchen, plus a broad selection of other merchandise such as greeting cards, children's toys, bathroom accessories, candles and gifts. I opened my store in a small space on a shoestring budget and hired only one employee, Jo. The two of us opened the doors of the store in November of 1982. Even though I knew very little about operating a retail store, *Kitchens Plus* was a big hit and soon became known as Manhattan's "fun place to shop."

Kitchens Plus started in only 1,200 square feet of space. A year later, I expanded to 2,500 square feet and the following year, I moved the store across town into 5,000 square feet of space and added a small café in the middle of the store. *The Croissant Café* had only four tables and counter space for six, but managed to do a brisk business selling fresh-baked croissants, homemade soups, desserts and fresh ground coffee.

In early 1986, a huge 12,000-square-foot space became available next door to the busiest grocery store in town. I decided to move and expand my store again. I signed a five-year lease and spent almost my entire savings to remodel the space and expand my café to accommodate 100 diners.

In less than four years, *Kitchens Plus* had grown from one of the smallest stores in town into one of the largest with a staff of 14 employees. My store had definitely become "the place" to shop or to enjoy a delicious lunch or a piece of homemade cheesecake and a cup of coffee. I often joked that *Kitchens Plus* was the top tourist attraction in town. Almost everyone who had out-of-town company brought their visitors into *Kitchens Plus* to shop and enjoy a cup of coffee or lunch in *The Croissant Café*.

During the first part of 1986, I was exhausted from the move but expected my life would soon slow down. I loved the new and expanded *Kitchens Plus*. I looked forward to having time to concentrate on keeping my customers happy and providing them with one of the best places in town to shop and have fun. All that changed later that year after I learned Jim was dying from complications of AIDS, and that Scott and I were HIV-positive.

At first, I was terrified I would die within two years. After all, that was Dr. Wade's prediction. I had just signed my five-year lease agreeing to pay $7,500 per month in rent for my store and restaurant. The rent, utilities and taxes due for the next five years totaled nearly half a million dollars! Distressed, I picked up the phone and nervously called my landlord and informed him that I had just been diagnosed with "a terminal disease" and asked, under the circumstances, if there was any way I could shorten or cancel my lease? His response, *"I'm so sorry, but absolutely not!"*

After discussion with a lawyer, I learned that even death does not cancel a commercial lease. If I died while the lease was in force, the landlord would have the right to go after my assets to collect whatever part of the half million in rent I still owed. The news was devastating, especially since I was already worried about the financial impact my illness and death would have on my sons, Matt and Chris.

As if my health and impending death were not enough to worry about, I also was terrified that someone in Manhattan would learn I was infected with HIV. In 1986, virtually everyone was afraid of anyone with HIV/AIDS. At that time, many people thought you could catch the disease as easily as the common cold, simply by being in the room with someone who was infected, drinking out of their glass or from a cough or a sneeze. I was convinced that if word got around town that I had HIV, I would come to work one day, unlock the doors and not a single customer would walk in to shop or have lunch. I would be bankrupt within weeks. My fears were not unfounded. In 1986, even many in the medical profession were afraid to treat anyone with HIV.

I knew that if word leaked out that I was HIV-positive, my store and café would never survive. But I had to tell someone. I desperately needed someone to talk to. There was no way I could handle it by myself. However, I knew I could only tell people I trusted completely to keep their mouths shut and not tell anyone.

My partner at the time, Scott, obviously was aware of my HIV status, and he was as concerned about keeping the "news" from the public as much as me. If my memory is correct, the first person I shared my positive status with, after Scott, was my best friend, Dennis; the second person was Debbie, my sister. Debbie is only 21 months younger, and we've always been extremely close. When I went away to college at KSU, Debbie followed me two years later. After graduating, both of us decided to stay in Manhattan and did so for more than 20 years. Telling Debbie I was HIV-positive was a heartwarming, tearful experience for us both. Here's my "baby sister" in her own words:

A note to my big brother

You asked, "Tell me what you felt like when I told you I was HIV-positive," or was it, "Tell me what you thought when I got sick." I know the reason it has taken me so long to put this on paper is because I knew it would be emotional for me.

I wonder if that surprises you. These emotions come from loving you so much and wanting you to know the depth of those feelings. So before I answer the question about how I felt when you got sick, first let me share another memory with you.

It is the memory of when you first told me you were gay. We were in front of your house on Ratone walking down the sidewalk. You seemed so distressed. I guess you were afraid of how I would react to the news. I can't remember if you were holding my hand or if you had your arm around me. I just remember somehow, we were touching. Maybe it was just shoulder-to-shoulder with our heads together. You said, "I have something I need to tell you. I want you to know I'm gay."

I don't think that revelation really fazed me much. I mean, you're my big brother; I love you. Why would that news even affect how I feel about you? Were you afraid I wouldn't love you? How could that news possibly alter my feeling for someone who had shared my childhood, who watched over me and always wanted what was best for his baby sister. I just remember us being close. I don't even remember us fighting much. Did we fight? Either way, you just always seemed to be there. So, there I was for you, hoping you knew that no matter what lay ahead, I would love you still.

And now, the question, which still remains, "How do I feel about your HIV status and the realization that this monster could somehow take my big brother away?"

Well, I just never believed that was possible. Some would call it denial. I call it faith. Even when you became sick, I knew you were going to be OK. And for the most part, I think you have been. Not that life has always been easy, but you persevered and made sure there was a reason to keep living. There was too much in life you still needed to do.

Perhaps there is always that little twinge of fear that you might get sick and die, but so far, I have to believe the faith is more powerful than the fear. Maybe it is just too painful to think about losing someone you love, so you just keep believing that nothing bad will happen and God answers that prayer. I think He meant for you to share your story with others so that maybe they could have a better, healthier, longer life. I prayed for you.

My heart told me that this disease would not take you. For you it would be different. How could you possibly not be here? You're my big brother.

I love you! – Debbie

Other than Scott, Dennis and Debbie, only two other people initially learned of my HIV status: Jo, my store manager who helped open *Kitchens Plus*, and LeAnne, my other store manager.

When I met Jo, she was in her mid-60s, stood about 4'8" tall and had what can only be described as a short gray Afro. Forgive me for being politically incorrect, but my nickname for her, which I fondly called her on many occasions, was "Midget." What Jo lacked in size, she definitely made up for in attitude. She was feisty, often "bossy" (especially when it came to bossing me around), and definitely not afraid to give anyone a piece of her mind. Jo was extremely protective of me (think "pit bull") especially after learning I had HIV. She was jealous of any female customers, employees or sales representatives that I happened to be "too" fond of. At times, it appeared Jo was even jealous of my mother. It was sometimes laughable and sometimes annoying.

There was no doubt Jo wished to be the "number one" woman in my life. It was as if someone crossed my mother with a jealous lover and the end-result was Jo. We had a love-hate relationship, but mostly love. We were friends for more than 25 years, before she passed away a few years ago.

My other store manager, LeAnne, became, and remains one of my closest friends. Her daughter, Ashley, was nearly born in the front seat of my brand new Honda Prelude. I distinctly remember speeding to the hospital while she was in labor. As I raced down the street, I screamed at LeAnne, *"Don't you **dare** let your water break in the front seat of my new car!"*

Message from LeAnne

When I met Don, I was in my early 20s. At that time in my life the closest I had been to someone with a life threatening illness was watching the news or reading an article about someone with cancer, diabetes or lupus. I felt empathy even though they were strangers.

When your close friend, who's been there for you through your highs and lows, tells you he's been diagnosed with HIV – Oh my God, not "that word" – the one said in fear on the news every night – you don't feel empathy.

I would describe the feeling as gut-wrenching, overwhelming sorrow. I NEEDED him in my life; he can't die – not now, not this way.

I love you Don, I'm so thankful that this disease has not taken your life, but instead has given you greater purpose – LeAnne Williams

By the end of 1986, Scott, Dennis, Jo, Debbie and LeAnne all knew I was HIV-positive. I shared my HIV status with only a few additional people during the next five years. It was five years before my parents, sons, brother and the majority of my other family members and close friends officially heard the news.

In the early part of 1986, I loved going to work every morning. I looked forward to every minute I was at *Kitchens Plus*. I loved interacting with my staff and customers. Life was fun!

The fun stopped in September 1986. I had HIV. Learning I was HIV-positive destroyed my eagerness to dash out the door every morning to head to the store. My daily joy and eagerness were replaced with never-ending apprehension of what the day would bring. Every morning for the next five years, whenever I unlocked the door to my businesses, I worried it might be the day when the words – "Don has AIDS" – leaked out and no one would shop at *Kitchens Plus* or eat in *The Croissant Café* ever again. Manhattan's "fun place to shop" would instantly be destroyed. AIDS would "kill" the business I loved – and then it would kill me.

When someone is HIV-positive, doctors typically want blood labs drawn every three months to determine how well the immune system is holding up and to check the progression of the virus. A few months after my diagnosis, Dr. Wade wrote an order for me to have some blood work done. I took the order into *Peterson Labs*, the main medical lab in Manhattan, to have blood drawn. When I walked into the waiting room, I saw four lab technicians, all of whom were regular lunch customers of *The Croissant Café*. Needless to say, I turned right around and drove home to call Dr. Wade and tell him there was no way I could ever have lab work done in Manhattan.

For the next five years, I drove 60 miles to Topeka anytime I needed to see the doctor, have any lab work or go to the pharmacy. I couldn't do any of those things in Manhattan, because almost everyone in town had been in my store or café at some point in time. I had to keep my condition a secret.

To be honest, I don't remember a lot about the first few years after Dr. Wade confirmed I was indeed infected with HIV. I buried myself in work, often putting in 12 to 14-hour days during the week and working most Saturdays and Sundays. When I was working, I could sometimes forget for at least a few hours that I had HIV. When I went home and was not working, I could rarely think of anything except the fact I was infected with HIV. I found myself having a drink as soon as I walked in the door. After downing the first drink, I would have another – and then another – eventually, drinking myself to sleep. The next day I would drag myself out of bed, go to work and put in another long day. Then I would repeat the process by driving home to drink myself into another stupor.

In addition to dealing with the fact I had what was considered at the time to be a fatal disease, I also was coping with the fallout and guilt experienced by many divorced fathers. Instead of seeing Chris and Matt every day and experiencing the joy of tucking them into bed every night like most fathers, the time I had to spend with my sons was "planned" and limited. Karen remarried a few years after our divorce and in 1985, the company she and her new husband worked for transferred them to Americus, Georgia.

Before my sons moved to Georgia with their mom, I saw them on Wednesday nights and every other weekend. It was depressing enough when I only saw Chris and Matt a few days a week before they moved out of state. After the move, my depression intensified since visits with them consisted of seeing them once or twice a year during a holiday and having them stay with me for about six weeks each summer. Even before my diagnosis with HIV, it was depressing to play the role of a "part-time" father and only see my sons a few times a year. It was also hard on Chris and Matt. Divorce is definitely not fair, especially for children who are only victims and are in no way responsible for the upheaval in their lives.

Once I learned I was infected with HIV and would likely die within a couple of years, my role as a father became pure agony. I felt as if I were literally torn in half. Part of me desperately wanted to spend as much time with Chris and Matt as possible to try to give them a lifetime of love in the few years that I had left. The other part of me wondered if it might be better to spend less time with them so they were not as emotionally attached to me. The last thing I wanted to do was to hurt them more. I was afraid the more time we spent together, the more fun we had and the more they loved me, the more they would hurt once I died.

I reached a point where I was in constant emotional pain – so much pain I actually ached physically. I missed Chris and Matt every day. My depression was almost unbearable, and the only way I could escape the pain was to stay busy at work during the day and drink myself to sleep at night.

When I did have the opportunity to see Chris and Matt over a holiday or during their summer vacation, it was impossible for me to completely enjoy their visit. I was torn between using our time together to develop and nurture a close, loving relationship or trying to not be so loved by them that my death would tear them apart. I was trapped in what felt like a no-win situation. Looking back, I feel I often failed as a father.

At the end of one of their summer visits, I hit rock bottom after putting Chris and Matt on a plane to fly back home. I left the airport in tears and began my two-hour drive back to Manhattan. As I drove, my sadness turned into despair. I had just dropped off my sons and would not be seeing them again until at least Christmas. My best friend, Dennis, had been steadily getting "crazier" and was going downhill quickly. In addition to Dennis, Kenny was sick and I had a couple of other friends with HIV who were starting to struggle with one health issue after another. As soon as I arrived home, I poured myself a glass of Scotch.

I was racked with guilt: guilt from getting a divorce and destroying my family, guilt from what I was putting my sons through and guilt from remaining healthy while my friends were dying. When I started drinking that night, I distinctly remember the bottle of Scotch was nearly full. I kept drinking and at some point I snapped. Life was no longer bearable. Suddenly it was clear what I had to do. The only way out was to kill myself. I went to the kitchen and grabbed the biggest knife I owned, a butcher knife.

I headed to the bathroom carrying the Scotch bottle in one hand and the butcher knife in the other. I planned to slit my wrists in the shower thinking it would be easier for someone to clean up the mess. I undressed, climbed in the shower and turned on the water – adjusting the temperature so it was barely warm. I sat down on the floor in the shower and lifted the bottle of Scotch to take another drink. The next thing I remember is waking up in the shower with the water running. The water was ice cold. I was lying on the floor in my tiny shower with an empty Scotch bottle in one hand, my butcher knife still in the other.

It is commonly said that those with drug or alcohol problems need to "hit bottom" before they have enough willpower to climb out of their addiction. There I was, literally lying in the bottom of my shower, naked and freezing. Dropping the bottle and knife, I struggled to my feet to turn off the water. I stepped out of the shower, grabbed a towel and fell to the floor sobbing. Eventually, I cried myself to sleep lying on the floor.

When I awoke, I realized I was at a turning point. I could either continue to use alcohol as a means to cope until it finally destroyed me, or I could take control my life. I was fed up and ashamed that I had used alcohol in an attempt to cope with the fact I was a divorced parent, who also happened to have a fatal illness. Lying on the floor that morning, I made myself a promise: *"I will not drink a single drop of alcohol for the next year."*

During the next 12 months, I did not have a cocktail, beer or glass of wine, not even a sip. I stopped drinking without the help of Alcoholics Anonymous or any other counseling. However, I did have help. I prayed. Anytime I had the urge to have a drink to kill the pain, I prayed.

In addition to praying, I began to focus daily on something my beloved grandmother, Nan, said to me repeatedly while I was growing up, **"Don, it doesn't do any good to worry about things you cannot change."** I could not change the fact that I was divorced and infected with HIV. However, I did not have to die in two years just because my doctor said it was "likely" I would. Just because my friends were dying did not mean I had to die as well.

No matter what anybody said, I was determined to live long enough to see Chris and Matt graduate high school in 10 years. I knew if I continued to drink heavily, I would never make it.

The years continued to creep by, and I remained healthy. But despite my new determination to remain in control of my life, it was never easy. The stress of watching my friends die from complications of AIDS was, at times, too much to bear. I was terrified anytime I discovered I had a new bruise or the slightest fever. Even though I continued to be in good health, I could not help but feel as if an "ax" was always hanging over my head. I wondered constantly when it would finally fall.

In addition to watching Dennis' mind and body literally deteriorate before my eyes, I had other friends with HIV/AIDS who were dying, like Kenny and Jon.

Jon was a school psychologist who loved his job. He worked with Down syndrome elementary and middle school students as well as other students with various developmental challenges. For several summers I had the pleasure of helping Jon coach his kids during the Special Olympics. Jon rented a small cottage that I owned, behind my house. We were constantly running back and forth between our two places to hang out together.

Jon **never** purchased any new clothes, furniture or household goods. He was a thrift store junkie. Virtually everything he owned came from a garage sale, a thrift shop and sometimes even the dump. One of my most cherished memories involving Jon is of five days we spent together driving his Volkswagen Rabbit from one side of Nebraska to the other. It was during the heat of the summer and Jon, who was at times a bit eccentric, invited me along for a thrift store adventure. His objective: spend five days driving from one end of Nebraska to the other in search of every thrift store in the state.

We left Manhattan one Monday morning, with the convertible top down, and headed north to Nebraska. After we crossed the state line, we headed west. Starting in the western part of Nebraska, we zigzagged north and south stopping in one small town after another so Jon could browse at each local thrift store. Every "junk store" (my term) where we stopped, Jon would dig through piles of "crap" (my term) and whoop with delight whenever he found a new "treasure" (his term).

For five days – it seemed like a lifetime to me – we were like a pinball bouncing around the hot, dusty state of Nebraska. Thankfully, the trunk quickly filled up with Jon's "treasures" and he finally turned on the air-conditioning after reluctantly closing the convertible top. With the trunk full, he began filling up the back seat from floor to ceiling with his new treasures. The last day of our trip, we arrived in Omaha on the east side of the state.

By the time we headed home the next morning, Jon's VW Rabbit was stuffed like a Thanksgiving turkey. Every square inch of the trunk and inside of the car was crammed with what I considered to be mostly trash. Jon beamed with delight. In five days, I purchased **one** item, an antique green glass jar with a lid. Today, more than 20 years later, that small jar sits on my kitchen counter filled with pistachios. Whenever I remove the lid, it brings back fond memories of Jon and our five-day thrift store junket.

Not long after our trek through Nebraska, Jon confided in me that he, too, was HIV-positive. I was stunned. How was it possible that another of my close friends had HIV? I wanted to run away – leave Manhattan. I could not bear the thought of watching another person I loved get sick and perish. I never wanted to see another friend of mine lying in a hospital bed in diapers.

After Jon died from complications of AIDS, I attended his memorial service in the *All Faiths Chapel* on the K-State campus. The night of the service, it was dark, cold and dreary. I was alone and sat near the front of the chapel. I was surprised; it seemed that very few people were there. I closed my eyes and silently said my good-byes to Jon. Desperately, I wanted to cry in hopes it would help relieve the depth of my pain. Try as I might, I could not. My heart ached to the point my entire body physically hurt. I knew I would miss my friendship with Jon immensely.

Dennis, Kenny and Jon were only a few of those I knew who contracted HIV and went on to die from AIDS. It was almost impossible for me to believe how many people I personally knew who were getting sick and dying. One day, in a rage, I threw away my address book. I could no longer stand to look up anyone's phone number. Whenever I did, I would stumble across a name or two scratched out because the person had died from the same disease I was living with every day.

Unbelievably, I stayed healthy from the time I tested positive in 1986 until the lease on my store expired in the fall of 1991. I was lucky enough that even though a few of my customers and friends may have started to suspect I might have HIV, they apparently cared enough not to share their suspicions with others. During 1991, my store was always busy with shoppers, as well as people dining in the café. My business was flourishing. *Kitchens Plus* and *The Croissant Café* were truly one-of-a-kind places, and the public loved them.

However, with my lease almost up, I felt as if I had no choice but to close. In the previous five years, I had been lucky enough to stay healthy. However, during those five years, I watched friends who were diagnosed with HIV about the same time as I was die.

The most difficult year of my life was 1991. To the dismay of thousands of my customers, I made the decision to close *Kitchens Plus* and *The Croissant Café* and move back to Kansas City. For the next four months, I went to work every day, pulled up in front of my business, only to be greeted by a huge "Going Out of Business" sign in the front window. On the final day of *Kitchens Plus'* existence, the last of the inventory, store fixtures and restaurant equipment were sold at auction. All day, I struggled to hold back tears and not break down in front of my friends and customers who came to say goodbye. As soon as the auction ended, I locked the door for the last time and climbed into my car. I sat at the wheel for a long time before I could turn the key. *Kitchens Plus* and *The Croissant Café* had been a huge part of my life. HIV robbed me of one of my most cherished dreams.

From Nancy Kiefer, a "regular" of Kitchens Plus

When my husband and I moved from Los Angeles to Manhattan, Kansas in 1982, I experienced culture shock! I will never forget the day I met Don and discovered his store, Kitchens Plus. The store was filled with wonderful, unique items that were attractively displayed and temptingly promoted. I felt absolute relief to find a place that resembled a piece of the "big city" life I had left behind.

Weekly visits to the store kept me energized, and well, sane. It didn't take long to realize that even more important than the store was the friendship we were forming with Don. His diverse life experiences, broad-minded perspective and positive approach toward life were invaluable to accepting Manhattan as home.

When I found out that Don was HIV-positive and he was closing his store, I was devastated. First and foremost, I was afraid I was losing a friend; even though Don promised to keep in touch, I wasn't sure that his medical diagnosis would allow for that. Also, visits to the store and its café had become a regular part of my family's Saturday activities.

Happily, today, we continue to share a wonderful friendship with Don. And, while there has never been another store like Kitchens Plus in Manhattan, I have some great memories of the times my family and I spent there. – Love, Nancy

Because I was moving to Kansas City, I also had to sell my house. Twelve years earlier, when I divorced, I moved from one of the nicest homes in town into a 70-year-old, dilapidated bungalow. I spent eight years transforming my rundown house into a cozy, updated home complete with a sunroom, hot tub and a beautifully landscaped yard. I hated to sell my home, but I had no choice. I was moving.

At the time, I had two affectionate and very spoiled housecats: Blackjack and Rassie. Once I moved to Kansas City, I planned to start a sales position requiring me to travel and felt it would be inhumane for my cats to be stuck at home alone for days at a time. On impulse, I gave Blackjack and Rassie to a couple I didn't even know. The couple had two children and Blackjack and Rassie were both terrified of children. I don't know what I was thinking, but I'm sure my beloved cats went on to have a horrifying life. Sometimes I wonder if they're waiting in the hereafter to claw me to death.

To top things off, the same month I closed my business, sold my home and abandoned my pets – I ended a three-year relationship.

Yes, 1991 was a horrible year. I loved my store, my house, my cats and all the many friends I had made in Manhattan since moving there 22 years earlier. Having HIV and the fear of eventually developing AIDS forced me to give up everything.

In late fall of 1991, I moved back to Kansas City where most of my immediate family still lived. It had been more than five years since the day I drove to Dr. Wade's office and learned I was infected with HIV. It had been more than five years since I had been told to *"get my affairs in order"* because I would be *"sick within a year and more than likely die within two."* But I was not sick. I was still alive and well. However, I felt as if closing my business, selling my home and moving closer to family were steps I had to take to *"get my affairs in order."* Many of my major dreams and goals had ended. I was returning to Kansas City to die.

"Get your affairs in order"

When I returned to Kansas City, I did not purchase another house. From the time I was old enough to push a lawn mower, I loved working in the yard. My professionally landscaped, perfectly manicured lawn in Manhattan had been my pride and joy. I could "lose myself" while mowing, pruning and trimming; I rarely thought about any of my problems while puttering around the yard. Working up a sweat and getting dirt under my fingernails was better therapy than money could buy.

Maintaining a lawn, at least to my picky standards, required a lot of time and effort. I feared that once my health started to deteriorate, the effort would be more than I could handle. Thus far, I had been lucky. I was still alive and had not been sick in five years. However, I couldn't expect my luck to continue. Soon, I would be sick and unable to take care of myself, let alone a lawn. The yard work I loved to do would become a burden, one that might fall upon the shoulders of my friends or family.

Instead of buying a house, I purchased a condo. I viewed it as taking one more step to *"get my affairs in order"* before my death.

Shortly after moving, I began work as a sales representative offering upscale, often imported children's toys, games and gadgets to specialty toy stores. Doing so required traveling a two-state territory. I hated it. I hated being on the road three or four days a week. I hated staying in hotels. I hated eating lousy food in dirty restaurants. I missed my friends. I missed my cats. I missed the daily hustle and bustle of retail. I was miserable.

As much as I hated my job, there was another step required to *"get my affairs in order"* that I dreaded far more. Since being diagnosed I had shared my status with only a handful of people.

No one in my immediate family, with the exception of my sister, Debbie, knew for sure I was infected. It was time to disclose my health situation to my family and loved ones, **before** I was sick, hospitalized and dying. It was time to tell my mom, dad and brother, Dave. Even more frightening, it was time to tell my sons. My oldest son, Chris, was now 16 and Matt had just turned 13. I knew they deserved time to adjust to my impending health challenges, and emotionally prepare for my death.

My parents and brother were obviously saddened by the news, but not totally surprised. All three of them had met Dennis and Kenny and knew from their appearance and hearing me talk, that both were dying of AIDS. Over the previous five years, my demeanor, no doubt, also provided some clues. Once they learned about my decision to close *Kitchens Plus,* all the clues fell into place. My family and closest friends knew I would have never made the decision to stop doing what I obviously loved doing without being forced to do so.

"Your dad has HIV"

Throughout my life, I have often felt fear, but rarely to the level I experienced when thinking about telling Chris and Matt that I was infected with HIV. Hadn't I hurt them enough? Through no fault of their own, they had been tiny victims of a broken home. Instead of living with a father who loved them more than life itself, they were prisoners of what I can only describe as a "wicked stepfather," one who while not physically cruel, was often verbally abusive.

As soon as I was settled after my move to Kansas City, I knew it was time to break the news. I dreaded doing so, but I wanted my sons to hear it from me before I was sick and in the hospital. They deserved time to process the news before the inevitable occurred. At the time, telling someone you had HIV was like saying, *"I'm going to die."* Desiring to minimize the emotional fallout as much as possible, I contacted a therapist specializing in family therapy to help me rehearse what to say. A few months later, when Chris and Matt arrived for their summer visit, the three of us went to the therapist's office where I planned to divulge my secret with the therapist at my side for moral support.

When we arrived, Matt and Chris knew "something was up." I was nervous and sweating profusely. How do you tell your 13 and 16-year-old sons that, in essence, you are going to die? How do you reveal you have a terminal illness without causing emotional heartache? I knew it was impossible.

Believe it or not, there is little about the actual disclosure I remember. Shock does wonders to help us deal with unbearable physical and emotional pain. I vaguely recall that both Matt and Chris appeared to take the news in stride. I remember shedding tears, but I am not sure if either of them did. Likely, they were in shock. Somehow, we ended up talking about Dennis even though it was definitely not in my plan to do so. When Chris and Matt were little boys, I often took them to Dennis' place in the country. Near his home was an old farm pond where Dennis loved to take them fishing. He taught my sons to put a worm on the hook, something I hated to do.

My sons loved fishing with Dennis, and we often visited him. As a result, I was not the only one who witnessed the deterioration of his mind and body. Chris and Matt were exposed to the decline of their fishing buddy's health. As things worsened, I tapered off their visits and finally stopped taking them to see Dennis. Even though they were spared from seeing Dennis bedridden, they knew he had AIDS. While it was not discussed directly while we were at the therapist that day, I'm sure that once they learned I had the same disease that killed Dennis, they were terrified.

A few months ago, I asked Matt, who is now 33, and Chris, who is now 35, to share some thoughts about what they remember about their teen years when told I had HIV, and what impact it has had on their lives.

Matt's thoughts:

When I was 13, my father told me that he was HIV-positive. It was a shock to say the least. It was the early nineties and what I knew about HIV at the time, I had learned in junior high health class. Basically I learned that if you get HIV you probably wouldn't live but a few years.

No one bothered to tell me that my father had already lived those few years, and a few more besides. If they had, I don't know if it would have made the situation better or worse.

It was stressful at first; I expected that any day could be the day I learned my father was sick and it was time to go say goodbye. And it wasn't the kind of thing you wanted to talk to your friends about at that age, so you just kept that fear inside.

It's been 20 years since then. I don't have the same feelings of impending doom as I did when I was a teenager, but from time to time those feelings come back, especially when Grandma calls with a false alarm.

Chris: My thoughts on having a dad with HIV

This is a hard topic for me to talk or write about because during most of my childhood I felt as if adults were trying to protect or shield me from the truth – that you were sick. Most of my childhood, I knew that something wasn't right because you were tired or didn't feel well or needed to rest, etc. But no one was ever honest about the reason why.

When you finally told us, all it did was confirm what I had been feeling for a long time. I felt cheated and angry that something I suspected for years was true.

Looking back on that time is very frustrating. A lot of my teenage life was spent thinking about how much do I tell people about my dad? What will they think? Will I lose them as a friend if they know? It wasn't until I got to college and figured out that other people's actions and opinions didn't matter much that I finally became comfortable talking about your life and that you had AIDS.

I think a lot of my uncertainty growing up was a direct result of how information was hidden from me as a child, and, in all honesty made me always second guess myself as a child.

I am through thinking about the past. I have moved on; I'm happy. I have a great wife, children, friends and family.

The comments from my sons leave me with overwhelming sadness. Growing up, Chris suspected that something was wrong and felt *"cheated and angry"* that he wasn't told about my HIV sooner. I'm not sure if I understand how those feelings led him to *"second guess"* himself while growing up, but the fact is that it affected his attitude about himself. Rather than trying to protect my oldest son from learning his father had a terminal illness, I should have confirmed what he suspected much earlier.

Another event that may have influenced Chris's self-image took place years earlier, when Karen and I divorced. We learned months later that Chris, who was only four years old, blamed himself for me leaving. Many months after the divorce, Karen's mother, Barbara, who had just spent a few days with Chris, told us that he said, *"The reason my mom and dad got divorced was because I made too much noise."* I was heartbroken. Chris, who was only three when we separated, apparently had walked around for months believing he was to blame. How he drew the conclusion that his noise was responsible for our marriage ending, I have no idea. I certainly understand how carrying around the "blame" for breaking up our family may have had a lasting impact on his self-esteem.

Matt's comments are not quite as hard for me to swallow as those from Chris. However, it is disheartening to hear that even though I broke the news about my HIV status, I obviously "dropped the ball" by rarely talking about it after that. I didn't think about having any ongoing discussions to address their concerns during the remainder of their teenage years. Over the next 10 years, I rarely, if ever asked how they were doing. On the other hand, they frequently heard about most of the medical challenges I continued to face, often from a third party. Looking back, I should have been more attentive to their needs.

I have not been a perfect father. Hopefully, after reading this book, Chris and Matt will have a better understanding of the emotional trauma I endured on a daily basis after learning I had HIV. Hopefully, they will have a better understanding of why I felt as if conflicting forces were tearing me in half. Hopefully, they'll understand I did the best I could under the circumstances. Hopefully they never doubted that I loved them.

As a child, it is difficult to understand why a parent may or may not do what the child expects. As an adult, especially an older one, you begin to develop a better understanding about "why" someone you trusted to protect and love you, behaved in a certain way. Understanding "why" does not mean the action was correct. It simply means you start to grasp a sense of why parents do what they do, even when it is wrong and may seem unforgiveable.

"To h--- with getting my affairs in order"

After 18 months of despising my job, I was at wits end. One day, I had a conversation with my dad, telling him how I hated my job. It was not the least bit emotionally satisfying, and I desperately missed the interaction and fun I enjoyed with past customers, many of whom had become good friends.

Dad suggested that I do what I loved to do and open another store. I explained the reason I had closed *Kitchens Plus* was because I was worried that when the inevitable happened and I finally developed AIDS, I wouldn't be able to work, let alone manage a business with other employees. Opening another store would definitely not be taking a step to *"get my affairs in order."* I did not want to put myself in a position that would eventually create an uncertain future for my employees and a financial disaster for my family.

Dad proposed I go into partnership with Jonni, his second wife's niece. At the time, Jonni was in her 20s and had not yet found her career niche. My dad suggested that I train Jonni, who had little business experience, so she would be capable of taking over the primary management duties if my health started to fail.

During the next few weeks, after much discussion and serious thought, I decided to open up *Kids Plus Me*. I set about finding a location and designing what would be the most colorful, fun-filled store in Kansas City. My concept: A toy store for young shoppers of all ages and a gift shop for their moms. The inventory would include upscale, educational toys as well as gifts, books and clothing for children. In addition, the store would have a unique selection of gifts carefully chosen to appeal to the moms who most often shopped with or for their children.

Besides having Jonni as a partner in the venture, my mother, Shirley, readily agreed to work part-time. It seemed to be a perfect solution. Since *Kids Plus Me* was a smaller retail store and did not include the many headaches associated with owning a restaurant, it was a more manageable undertaking than my previous business. I also had Jonni and my mom to rely on for help if necessary. I signed a three-year lease, and the store opened in the fall of 1993.

<u>Thoughts from my mom, Shirley</u>

It is very hard for me to explain how I felt when you told me about being infected with HIV. My first emotion was disbelief that this could be happening to my beloved son. And then I was angry, scared, devastated and all the other emotions that go with this type of news.

I took some comfort in the fact you decided to move back to K.C. after being gone for 22 years. I thought at least I could be there with you and help you when you needed it.

The more you lost friends to this disease the harder it was. You live with such fear and uncertainty at a time like this. I tried a support group with people who had HIV or had lost loved ones. I found it so depressing that I had to quit going.

At that time, they did have one doctor speak who said that someday they hoped there would be treatment for AIDS and it would be more of a chronic illness like diabetes, but at that time there wasn't much medication to do that. He said that testing of drugs was on a 'fast track.' That at least gave me hope that you would be able to get medicine to treat the disease.

When you decided to open Kids Plus, I was thrilled that I could work with you as it gave us precious time to spend together. I will always treasure that time, the fun we had and all the good things and people we met there.

Most people with HIV who lost as many friends as you did would just sit and wait to die. The most important thing you have done, as far as I'm concerned, is that you started telling your story to students in high schools and churches. I know your message has changed a lot of behavior and hopefully saved many lives.

I would have to say to you Don, how proud I have always been of you for your personal fortitude on days that I know you have not felt well but continue to spread your message by the kind of life you live. You have helped me realize how precious life is and how we can hopefully look back at our life and be proud of what we've done for others and that we are loved by our friends and family. I hope you will always know how much you are loved and admired.

Love always, Mom

In reality, I wasn't ready to throw in the towel and die. I quit the "job" I dreaded doing every day and went back to doing what I loved to do – providing a delightful place for people of all ages to shop and enjoy themselves.

At the same time I made the decision to open *Kids Plus Me*, I also decided to rent out my condo and buy another house. I hated condo life as much as I hated traveling with the trunk and backseat of my car packed full of toys. I missed my yard! I wanted a house and a lawn where I could putter around and forget for just a little while that I had HIV. So much for *"getting my affairs in order."*

Without going into detail, my partnership with Jonni failed to work out and we parted ways only a few months after opening *Kids Plus Me*. Suddenly, I was back in a situation similar to the one I had managed to free myself from when I closed my store and café two years earlier. I was again saddled with a three-year lease and a monthly rent payment to worry about. My old fear of getting sick and not being able to operate my business returned. At least I did have Mom to depend on. I knew I could always count on her.

For the next year, things were great. I loved being back in retail again. I loved working with new customers, who soon were shopping regularly in my store. I especially loved having many "young" shoppers. *Kids Plus Me* was the kid friendliest store in town, and shoppers of all ages were encouraged to enjoy themselves by "playing" while they shopped. I felt as if I had been reborn. I was having fun again. I loved going to work. But it would not last.

My life "crashed" and so did I

Starting in the beginning of 1995, I noticed "something" was changing. I went to work every day, but the abundant energy I was so accustomed to having seemed to stay at home. I found myself dragging around the store for what seemed to be ever longer, never-ending days. It was difficult, sometimes impossible, to put a smile on my face. Instead of enjoying my daily interactions with my young shoppers, I was starting to dread it. The little shoppers started getting on my nerves. I had frequent headaches. My first symptom of AIDS had arrived; I had HIV-related fatigue.

Crankier with each passing day, I started to snap at my employees, especially my mother. I had no energy to complete a task. When my staff or my mom attempted to do something that I normally focused my time and talent on accomplishing, it was never "done right." There were many days when I was absolutely mean to Mom, which only made me feel worse. I have no excuse other than my health, my life, was deteriorating rapidly. I knew my time to die was finally coming and I was angry. I took much of that anger out on my mother. Looking back, I'm sure I did so because I knew I could get away with it. Mom would love me no matter what.

Often I was so tired by lunchtime that I would collapse on the floor of my office to nap. Soon, I was only able to work half days and headed home immediately after Mom and the other members of my staff finished their lunch break. Once home, I crashed on the sofa for the remainder of the day.

One day in September of 1995, I felt especially lousy and went home after only working for a couple hours. I woke up on the sofa later that afternoon with a fever of 105 and ended up in the emergency room of Saint Luke's Hospital in Kansas City, Missouri. After seeing the doctor, I learned I had PCP, the most common cause of death for people with AIDS. It was the same disease that had taken my best friend, Dennis.

My CD4 count was zero, which indicated my immune system was no longer functioning. I was no longer a person infected with HIV; I had just progressed to someone with full-blown AIDS.

My "best buddy," Brad

I had a message in September 1995, "Don is in the hospital." Don had been diagnosed with Pneumocystis pneumonia – the dreaded opportunistic infection that meant full-blown AIDS. So many others had succumbed to this before him. Don had lost a great deal of weight and definitely had that gaunt look. I remember going to Saint Luke's Hospital in Kansas City on that September evening afraid of what was happening to my friend.

The hospital bed seemed to swallow him up and several IVs were pumping who-knows-what in an attempt to save his life. We kept the conversation light-hearted and if I remember right, Don was still able to muster a smile. We left there and I said, "I don't think he'll make it to Christmas." He looked that bad.

On a subsequent visit he wanted to take a shower. I helped him into the shower stall and was shocked by the decimated look of his body. It was skin and bones like a picture of someone out of a concentration camp.

Over the course of 12 days in the hospital we went back to check on his progress. One day he mentioned a dream he had and when he got out, he wanted to go to schools and educate kids about AIDS and how to avoid HIV. Little did we know that's exactly what he would do! That dream would become his passion to live. (And a little dog, Maggie, would help too, but that's another story.) – Brad Johnson

As I lay in the hospital, I was not afraid of dying. In fact, I was "ready to die." Physically, I was a mess, but emotionally, I had already accepted the fact I was going to die. I was actually relieved my emotional and physical struggle with this disease was almost over. I was in a reflective, peaceful and somewhat cheerful mood. I had been luckier than most.

Everyone I knew who had been diagnosed with HIV around the same time as I had passed away years earlier. I stayed healthy long enough to see my oldest son, Chris, graduate from high school and start college at Purdue University. My youngest son, Matt, was in his senior year and would be graduating in six months. God had come very close to answering my prayer to live long enough for my sons to complete high school.

Thanks to my after-death visit from Dennis, I wasn't afraid of dying and I was ready to face my own death. I was tired of living life wondering when the "ax" hanging over my head would fall.

One night, while I was asleep in the hospital, I had a dream. In my dream it was as if I were floating in huge, puffy white cloud. Even though I was alone, I felt protected, safe and loved. I was smiling, starting to drift off to sleep when suddenly I heard a forceful, yet gentle, voice. I was given a message, *"Don, I'm sorry but you're not going to die now. You still have a job to do. You're going to go out and teach teenagers what they need to know so that they never get AIDS."*

I woke up immediately. It had been a short dream, but I instantly knew my life was going to change. I was going to leave the hospital. I wasn't going to die anytime soon. I somehow knew the messenger in my dream did not intend for me to talk to a few teenagers. I knew I was going to be talking to hundreds and hundreds of them. I absolutely did not want to go out in the world and talk to people about AIDS. Public speaking was not something I enjoyed doing. However, I understood I did not have a choice in the matter. It was a "fact." I was going to teach teens and young adults about HIV/AIDS, to help prevent them from becoming infected.

I had spent the last 10 years preparing myself to die, and I was ready. After my dream, I was disappointed and almost angry. If I wasn't going to die, it meant I had to go back to living every day with that "ax" still hanging over my head.

When my best friend, Dennis, died of PCP in 1988, there was no effective treatment available to combat this nearly always-fatal opportunistic infection. Fortunately, by the time I was diagnosed with PCP, medical professionals had discovered that a drug called pentamidine, when administered intravenously, was effective in helping those with PCP. Once on pentamidine, my health started to improve, and within a couple of weeks, the doctor started to talk about releasing me from the hospital.

Each of us can recall certain "defining" moments of our life — events that mark what happened at a specific time in life or events that seriously impacted our lives. My marriage, my divorce, my HIV test, my "dream" are only a few of the defining moments in my life. While I was hospitalized with PCP, there was another defining moment in my life. It occurred one night when my dad came to visit.

I remember very little about the first week I was hospitalized. My fever was so high I was delirious at times. Even after my fever dropped, pain medication and drugs to combat PCP were continuously pumped into my system, so I was "out of it." When released, I was amazed to learn of the number of people who stopped by to see me and to say, what many assumed would be their *"goodbyes."* I have no recollection of ever seeing or speaking with most of those who dropped in to visit that week. Chris and Matt made an eight-hour trip from Indianapolis to Kansas City, and I barely can recall their visit. However, I distinctly remember my dad's visit, or at least I remember what happened when it was over.

Before leaving that night, my dad, shaking slightly and with tears in his eyes, bent down, gave me a hug and said, *"I love you."* For some of you, it might seem like a normal response from a father whose son was near death. For me, it was a defining moment. That evening was the first time in my life that I can recall my father giving me a hug and uttering those three simple words.

It is extremely difficult for my father to share his feelings with anyone. Growing up, I was taught that men never showed any emotion that might indicate weakness, and regardless of the circumstances, "men **never** cried." My dad was strict, not unlike many men of his generation. He was quick to express anger and disappointment, and rarely offered a word of praise. As a young child, I did not understand his frequent angry outbursts. As a teenager, I still could not understand. Even after entering adulthood, I could not understand.

Now, as an older adult, I have a better understanding. My parents married at a young age. My father turned 18 only a month before I was born. By age 22, he had a wife and three children to support. Can you imagine what it must have been like to have the responsibility of providing a home, clothing and food for a family of five at that age? It is easy for me to imagine my father angry, "trapped" in a situation he could do nothing about.

Reading my son Chris's comments with regard to *"second guessing"* his actions and beliefs while growing up is especially painful, because they remind me of my own feelings as a child. Feelings I never wanted my own children to experience.

Like my son, I second-guessed myself during childhood. My self-esteem was low; I doubted my self-worth and often felt like a failure. As I entered adulthood, my early professional success resulted because I worked hard to avoid failure, not because I wanted to achieve success. My sense of impending failure intensified after I left my marriage.

As a child, I feared showing any negative emotion, especially anger or disapproval. As an adult, I have learned that the expression of feelings is natural and necessary to maintain good physical and mental health. My ability to express my true emotions blossomed once my health failed, and I came face-to-face with my own mortality while still a young man. Since that time, I have survived a number of life-threatening illnesses. Most people are not forced to face death until later in life and once they do, the need to express their feelings before it is "too late" may take on a sense of urgency.

Over the years, my dad has mellowed. Like many men of his generation, he has feelings, but is not comfortable expressing them. Sharon, my dad's wife, shared a story with me about the time she and my dad went to the theater to see, *"Philadelphia,"* a film about a young successful attorney, played by Tom Hanks, who had Kaposi's sarcoma, an AIDS-related cancer. In the middle of the movie, my dad started to cry, got up, left the theater and refused to return to watch the rest of the film.

I asked Dad a number of times if he would like to write down any thoughts about how my HIV status has affected his life and was not surprised that he was unable to do so. After I asked him one last time if he had anything he wanted to share, he said, *"Just tell them, I said you're a good son."*

My father loves me, and no doubt always has. I believe that once he realized that I was at death's door, the need to express his love won out over the fear to do so. I'm thankful that my father's ability to show his feelings toward me has improved.

Stop and ask yourself, *"If I knew for a fact I would die tomorrow, is there anyone I want to say 'I love you' to before I go?"* Or do you need to clear your conscience by saying, *"I'm sorry"* to someone in your life? If so, today is the day to do this. As someone who has faced death, I can assure you that tomorrow may never come.

The AIDS Quilt

A month or two before I was hospitalized with PCP, a group of friends and I made plans to go see the NAMES Project AIDS Memorial Quilt, a portion of which was going to be displayed at the Municipal Auditorium in Kansas City. If you have never had an opportunity to see the AIDS Memorial Quilt, I strongly encourage you to do so. Seeing it is a sobering experience, one that brings nearly everyone who views it to tears.

The AIDS Quilt was started in 1985 to pay tribute to those who had lost their lives to AIDS. Each quilt panel is three feet by six feet, the approximate size of a human grave. The panels memorialize the life of a person lost to AIDS and are hand-made by friends and loved ones. Eight panels are sewn together to create a 12 foot by 12 foot section of the Quilt. If displayed on the floor, the sections of the Quilt are separated by enough space for those viewing them to be able walk around the individual sections to easily see each panel.

The entire AIDS Quilt was first displayed October 11, 1987, on the National Mall in Washington, D.C. From the time the first panel was completed in 1985, the number of panels had grown to 1,920, and covered a space larger than a football field.

One year later, the Quilt was displayed on the Ellipse in front of the White House. The size of the AIDS Quilt had increased four-fold to 8,288 panels and covered an area the size of four football fields. Friends, family, celebrities and politicians read aloud the names of each of the more than 8,000 people memorialized on the panels displayed.

Four years later, in 1992, the AIDS Quilt returned to Washington where the display covered an area the size of 25 football fields. The last display of the entire Quilt was in Washington in October 1996. It is doubtful that the AIDS Quilt will ever be seen again in its entirety. It is now simply too large to display in any one place. As of March 2010, there were 91,000 panels with a total weight of 56 tons. If you were to spend only one minute viewing each of the 91,000 panels, it would take you 33 days to see the entire Quilt.

When the AIDS Quilt exhibit opened in Kansas City, I was stuck in my hospital bed, hooked up to an IV pumping pentamidine through my veins. My pneumonia was getting better, but was not gone. Knowing the Quilt was only going to be in Kansas City for three days I was determined to see it. My doctor had mentioned I might be well enough to go home on Tuesday, but the exhibit was leaving the Sunday before. After practically demanding to be released in time to go see the AIDS Quilt, my doctor reluctantly agreed to let me leave the hospital on Sunday afternoon.

Three of my friends, Jim, Paul and Brad, arrived at Saint Luke's to pick me up about lunchtime. I had lost 50 pounds and weighed only 119 pounds even though I was nearly six feet tall. Unable to walk, I left the hospital in a wheelchair with an oxygen tank attached. With the help of my friends, I climbed into the front seat of the car with my oxygen tank sitting on the floorboards between my feet. My wheelchair was loaded into the trunk, and we headed directly to the auditorium to see the AIDS Quilt.

Even though I felt lousy, I was ecstatic to be out of the hospital and on my way to see the Quilt. Two of my good friends, Ruth and Dean, whom I had known for 25 years, were volunteering at the exhibit that day, and I knew I would have a chance to see them. Ruth and Dean lived in Topeka and were like a second set of parents to me. They had three sons, John, Dean and Bob, who all attended K-State at the same time I did. The four of us were fraternity brothers. John, their oldest son, was one of my best college buddies and my best man when I married Karen.

After graduating from K-State, John's younger brother, Dean, moved to New York City and began a career as an artist. Regrettably, Dean contracted HIV sometime in the 1980s, and by 1991 was gravely ill from a number of AIDS-related complications. Ruth and Dean flew to New York and stayed for months to care for their son and help with his roommate, Bobby, who also had recently developed full-blown AIDS. Bobby died from complications of AIDS in September 1991, and Dean passed a month later.

Dean and Ruth always have had a strong Christian faith and attend church regularly. Ruth recently shared with me that after Dean died she *"was mad at God"* and *"stayed mad for a long time."* Since Dean's death, his parents have had an active role in HIV/AIDS prevention, been very involved in PFLAG (Parents, Families and Friends of Lesbians and Gays) and frequently volunteer to help whenever part of the AIDS Quilt is on display in the area.

When I arrived at the Municipal Auditorium that Sunday afternoon, we pulled up to the curb in front of the main entrance. My wheelchair was pulled out of the trunk and I settled into it with my oxygen tank on the seat beside me. My friends pushed me in the door.

When Ruth first caught a glimpse of me, she was overwhelmed by my appearance. Pale as a ghost, she bent down to greet me with a hug and a kiss. Years later, Ruth told me that on that day, she *"had a sinking feeling … like she was about to lose one more of her kids."* Dean said he looked at my emaciated body in the wheelchair and thought, *"I knew it was you in that chair, but at the same time it wasn't you."*

As I mentioned earlier, viewing the AIDS Quilt is a very somber experience. There are always plenty of tissues available and few people talk, and if they do, it is in a whisper. My friends slowly pushed me around that afternoon, stopping so I could read each panel on display. I was concentrating on the panels, when I realized that the people there that day were not only looking at the panels on the floor, but also were staring at me. I was in a wheelchair, breathing from an oxygen tank and so thin that I looked as if I had just been released from a concentration camp. As I passed others at the exhibit, I noticed many were uncomfortable making eye contact. Others would look directly into my eyes and give me a weak, yet friendly, smile.

Without intending to do so, my attendance at the AIDS Quilt added a completely new dimension to the experience. There I was, somewhere between a healthy living human being – and just another AIDS Quilt panel on the floor. That night on the news, the story about the AIDS Quilt included footage showing the back of a man in a wheelchair, a man who was obviously seriously ill. The identity of the man in the chair was not broadcast, but I knew I had made the news.

Another comment from my "best buddy," Brad

The AIDS Memorial Quilt was showing at the Music Hall the same weekend Don got out of the hospital. On a Sunday afternoon we took Don in a wheelchair to see this tribute to the many souls that had lost their battle. The exhibition hall was filled with quilts and the mood was somber. Don saw a couple from Topeka that came to see the Quilt of their son who had died of AIDS. Another reminder of the tragic loss caused by this disease.

Hard to believe Don not only survived, but also thrived since that bout of pneumonia. There would be other health scares to come along but he managed to navigate his way back to living. He is truly an inspiration. – Brad Johnson

There happened to be a volunteer at the AIDS Quilt exhibit that day who did not know who the sickly man in the wheelchair happened to be. However, there was no doubt in his mind that the person in the chair had full-blown AIDS and, more than likely, would have his own quilt panel one day soon. **Ironically, although neither of us knew it at the time, we were destined to meet.**

Life after PCP

When I started pentamidine IV treatment in the hospital, I soon learned that one of the side effects of the drug could be a sudden drop in blood pressure when going from a sitting or lying position to a standing one. In my case, the drop in blood pressure was so severe, and so sudden, that when I stood, I fainted. While hospitalized, on three different occasions, I attempted to get out of bed to go to the bathroom. Within a second or two of standing, I fainted, fell to the floor and awoke with a nurse or two "dragging" my body back into bed. After being politely threatened with "restraints," I agreed not to make another attempt to get up without calling a nurse for assistance.

After going home from the hospital, I continued IV treatments of pentamidine administered by a home healthcare nurse who came to see me several times a day. I quickly learned how to get to the bathroom and anywhere else I wanted to go without fainting. The solution was quite simple; I crawled on my hands and knees.

For the next couple of months while finishing pentamidine treatments, I crawled to the bathroom, crawled to the kitchen and even crawled outside to get the newspaper. Just before I was hospitalized, I hired a lawn service to kill off all the unwanted, miscellaneous grasses and weeds in my yard and reseeded the lawn. It needed to be watered daily. For weeks, I crawled around my yard moving around the sprinkler. My neighbors thought I was nuts.

When my treatments were finally finished, my PCP was gone. However, I still had full-blown AIDS and a CD4 count of zero. Basically, I had no functioning immune system. Realistically, I expected it would only be a matter of time before another opportunistic infection would appear and end my life.

Just in time, two critical events occurred after I was released from the hospital. I sincerely believe that without both events, I would not be alive today. While I was in the hospital, "the messenger" had given me a job to do, one I would never complete unless I not only survived, but also somehow found the strength to start knocking on the doors of a lot of high schools. Whether or not "the messenger" was directly responsible for these two events or not, I'll never know. But the timing was perfect, so I'll always wonder.

The first event took place in the spring of 1996, within a few months after my bout with PCP. The FDA approved the first protease inhibitor, a new class of drugs to fight HIV. I started taking a new "drug cocktail," which consisted of a protease inhibitor and two older HIV medications. Within a few months, my immune system took a turn for the better. My CD4 count of zero inched its way up to the low 200s. Not significant, but enough of an improvement that it appeared "the messenger" had arranged for me to have some additional time.

In my heart, I'm convinced that the second event is the real reason the "ax" has yet to fall. I'm still living because Maggie saved my life.

Maggie was six weeks old, weighed barely two pounds and was one adorable puppy. And I do mean adorable. Maggie appeared at my door one day in the hands of Anita, a young woman I had only known for a short time. As I opened the door, Anita smiled at me and exuberantly blurted, *"I brought you a present."*

Before even asking Anita to come in, I replied, *"You must be kidding. I can't even take care of myself. There's no way I can take care of a puppy."* Anita walked in the door and handed me Maggie. Grinning from ear to ear, she replied, *"That's exactly why I thought about giving her to you. You need something to worry about besides yourself."*

Apparently, Maggie's mother, not having much of a moral upbringing, was not a lady, but a tramp. Her mother was a medium-sized mutt – apparently a mix of yellow Lab, cocker spaniel, beagle and who knows how many other breeds. What about Maggie's father? No one had a clue about him. He apparently made an appearance and left, never to be seen again.

Anita shared that she had rescued Maggie from a family who needed to get rid of a litter of puppies immediately. One look into Maggie's big brown eyes, and I was hooked. She looked exactly like a Lab puppy, her coloring, as white as newly fallen snow. For a few brief hours, I even considered calling her Snowball. Then fate stepped in. About an hour after Maggie "moved in" and Anita left, my friend, Pat, stopped by to check and see how I was feeling. After seeing my new puppy, he offered to drive me to the pet store to pick up some necessities. On our way into the store, we passed a father carrying a little girl with a beautiful head of naturally curly brown hair. As soon as the little girl caught a glimpse of my new puppy, she excitedly proclaimed, "Doggy" and reached for the tiny pup.

The darling little girl tugged at my heart. She was one of the most beautiful toddlers I had ever seen. Her name was Maggie. Suddenly without thought, I asked her if she liked my puppy. She rapidly shook her head up and down, her brown curls shaking violently. I smiled and said, *"She likes you, too. In fact, she likes you so much she wants to know if it would be OK if I named her Maggie after you?"* If we had not bumped into Maggie and her father that day, poor Maggie would have been stuck with the name Snowball. That would have been a horrible name for a dog, especially since as she grew her coloring darkened to that of a yellow lab. If she were Snowball, she would have definitely been a dirty one.

Earlier, I mentioned that two events occurred just in time to save my life; I am quite sincere in this belief. The introduction of new HIV medications slightly improved my physical health. The introduction of Maggie into my life resulted in something I believe was even more vital. Maggie improved my emotional health. Her constant love and attention gave me a reason to live.

I went from life in a toy store with constant interaction with people of all ages to life at home alone. I talked to Maggie aloud as if she was human and she listened. Her understanding of words was amazing. At any one time, her toy box contained 10 to 15 different toys and on demand, she would dig through the box and return with the specific toy I requested. If she was given a new toy, I could repeat what it was called two or three times and she would remember the name.

When I recovered enough to show up at *Kids Plus Me* for a few hours a day, Maggie always went along. She loved playing with the young shoppers and they loved running around the store with Maggie at their heels. Maggie's favorite game was hide-and-seek. Believe it or not, she understood the rules.

Many of us love our pets. But few of us can make the claim their pet saved their life. I know Maggie saved mine. In those crucial months after my bout with PCP, she needed me, and I needed her. Maggie was my salvation.

<u>Anita's thoughts:</u>

The thing I remember the most about when Don told me he was "sick" is thinking, "Oh my God – he is going to die!" I didn't know him that well at the time and I wanted to spend as much time with him as possible in case he didn't have much time left.

Don has always said that Maggie saved his life and I believe that is true. It always helps knowing that someone or something needs you, and that makes you stronger. I'm just happy he is still here! He will probably out live all of us!

Time to tell my story

It was two or three months before I was well enough to leave the house for more than a short time. While recovering, I thought constantly about my dream and its message to educate teenagers about HIV. I lay in bed for weeks and wondered what I was supposed to do.

By nature, I wasn't a public speaker. In fact, I vividly remembered being terrified of any class in high school or college that required me to give a presentation to a group of people. I had no idea how to describe in words, in a short period of time how dramatically HIV impacted all aspects of everyday life. I had no experience talking to others about HIV/AIDS and even more discouraging, I had no credentials. After spending months trying to figure out what to do and how to do it, I realized I would never get any experience or credentials until I hauled myself out of bed and did something about it.

After much thought, it dawned on me to approach the principal of Shawnee Mission North High School in Mission, Kansas, a suburb or Kansas City. I graduated from Shawnee Mission North and was optimistic about the possibility that my own high school would be willing to let an alumnus speak. I parked in front of the school, went to the office and asked to speak to the principal. The principal's assistant inquired about why I wanted to see the principal, but I was too embarrassed to tell her I had AIDS or why I was there. I simply replied, *"It's personal."*

My conversation with the principal was brief. I introduced myself as an alumnus. I explained I had been living with HIV for 10 years, and had recently been diagnosed with AIDS. As soon as I mentioned AIDS, she drew back in her chair and tightened her grip on the armrest. Her discomfort with my presence was painfully apparent.

Before I ever entered the principal's office I was apprehensive. After her reaction to my health status, I knew I *"didn't have a chance"* of telling my story to the students at my alma mater. I awkwardly went on to explain that I was interested in speaking with the Shawnee Mission North students in hopes of preventing them from placing themselves at risk for HIV. Being honest, I disclosed the fact I had not yet had the opportunity to talk about my life with HIV and

AIDS to others, but believed that returning to my alma mater would be the perfect place to start.

The principal abruptly declared, *"I'll think about it"* and immediately arose from her chair to indicate our conversation was over. She backed away as she stood and motioned toward the door. It was obvious that she was genuinely fearful of being in my presence. I wrote down my contact information and left her office. Our entire conversation lasted two or three minutes. As I left, I had a suspicion the slip of paper with my name and phone number would end up in the trash before I left the building. Needless to say, I never received a call from the principal of my old high school.

My first attempt at carrying out my mission had failed. I had fallen flat on my face. I was depressed. If I couldn't convince the principal of my own high school to let me speak to students about HIV/AIDS, how would I ever convince anyone?

Four years before I developed PCP, I joined a small HIV/AIDS support group. There were eight members. We met weekly to talk, complain and sometimes cry. We shared feelings about how depressing it was to have one illness after another. We discussed the cost and debilitating side effects of the medications we were taking. We helped each other cope with the depression and financial woes that resulted when someone in the group had to give up his career because he was no longer healthy enough to work. During the first year of our support group, two of our eight members died from complications from AIDS.

Going to group every week was difficult, but it did help remind me that I wasn't alone in my struggles with HIV. Two social workers, Lydia and Rosalind, were wonderful women who facilitated group. Lydia and Rosalind volunteered two or three hours of their lives, every week, to help us deal with the physical, emotional and financial plights that continually confronted the members of our close-knit group.

One night during group, I told everyone about my dream in the hospital and how I "learned" of my mission to save others from HIV. My frustration was obvious, as I related the details of my prior visit with the principal of my former high school. I admitted that I thought the opportunity to talk to teenagers about HIV/AIDS would never materialize and I had no idea how to get my mission off the ground.

After I was through sharing, Rosalind said, *"Don, you can talk to my students."* As luck would have it, Rosalind was a school social worker who met frequently with two classes of at-risk high school students. I was ecstatic! Each class only had 10 to 15 students, but it was a start.

I don't recall if I did much preparation before I spoke to Rosalind's students. I know my initial presentation was anything but a canned speech. I simply sat at a table and had a conversation about my life. It wasn't difficult to do; I actually enjoyed myself.

Most of the students in Rosalind's class had a history of drug or alcohol abuse and almost all of them had been sexually active. I informally discussed how HIV could be transmitted by sharing needles when using drugs or by having sex without a condom. Talking about what it was like to watch my friends die, knowing I would more than likely follow in their footsteps, took up the most time.

Rosalind's students each wrote a letter thanking me for sharing such personal information about my life. Most mentioned that after hearing me talk about what it was like to have AIDS, and describing what my friends went through physically and emotional before their death had made a big impression in the way they thought about their future. None of them had any desire to contract HIV and after hearing my story, planned to be more careful in the future. When Rosalind gave me the evaluation letters, she included a reference letter expressing her enthusiasm about my impact on her students. The school's full-time social worker had also been present for my visit and Rosalind included a reference letter from her as well. Wow! I told my story to two groups of teenagers, and I was in possession of two reference letters. My journey had begun.

Over the next few years, with the help of those two reference letters, I gradually worked my way into more high schools. The number of reference letters grew from two to dozens, and word of my impact on students spread throughout the metropolitan area. My phone started ringing with requests to schedule presentations at high schools, colleges, church youth groups and numerous other organizations.

Initially, I spoke to individual classrooms of 20 to 25 high school students. The number of schools asking me to speak kept growing. Within a few years, I knew it would soon be impossible to speak to an ever-increasing number of individual classes. Having AIDS seriously limited my energy. After spending six or seven hours in a school speaking to one class after another, I was physically exhausted. In addition, the emotional drain repeatedly describing what it was like to watch Dennis and Kenny suffer and die took its toll.

One day I added up the number of presentations I had given during the month and was shocked to learn it was more than 100. I was at my physical and emotional breaking point. I had to make a dramatic change.

I implemented a new policy. Instead of telling my story to individual classes, I asked the teachers and school administrators to schedule an assembly, where I could tell my story to all the students studying HIV/AIDS that semester at one time. Most of the teachers and administrators understood my dilemma and agreed to my request. Rather than speaking to 20 or 30 teenagers in a classroom situation, I suddenly was telling my story to groups of 200 or 300 students at one time.

It seemed as if, out of the blue, I was a public speaker and it seemed easy. By speaking to larger groups, I was able to reach more people with my message at one time.

Starting in the early days of my mission, I kept count of the number of people who heard my story. I started my journey by talking to Rosalind's students in the fall of 1996, and stopped counting a number of years ago when the total number of those who had heard my story surpassed 100,000. While I don't charge a fee to speak to high school students, I always request evaluation letters from the students in the audience.

I have received thousands of letters. Some of them are only a paragraph long, but most of them are a page or two. Many writers believe I'm still alive because God wanted me to share my message with them. Whenever I read or hear this pronouncement, I think back to my dream in the hospital.

I have been HIV-positive for 30 years and have had AIDS for 15 years. Less than two percent of those infected with HIV in 1981, the year I believe I was infected, are still alive today. I am lucky to be alive. Many times I have wondered, *"Why am I still here?"*

Perhaps I really am still alive because God wanted me to tell my story to help teenagers and young adults not become infected with HIV.

A gift from "the messenger"

After my relationship with Scott ended, I re-entered the dating scene and eventually met Jim. We'd been together for about three years when I was hospitalized with PCP in the fall of 1995. Life with Jim was settled; we even owned a home together. While we were together as partners, I had HIV and Jim did not.

Serodiscordant couples, where one partner is HIV-positive and the other is HIV-negative, must take precautions to ensure the person who is HIV-negative stays that way. While it is possible to reduce the risk of HIV transmission drastically by practicing safer sex, sexual activity always contains some risk. It is understandable why this risk may result in stress for one or both parties in such a relationship.

Perhaps even more stressful than the anxiety resulting from a sexual relationship is the struggle that takes place if or when the infected person becomes seriously ill or dies. Being a caregiver and watching a loved one go through the death and dying process is not an easy task. It is equally difficult to be the one dying, watching someone you love forced into a position of helping you with the simplest and most basic human needs.

Even though Jim and I cared for each other a great deal, our sexual relationship was stressful. For the most part, we handled the strain fairly well. However, the stress in our overall relationship accelerated once my health started to deteriorate.

While a senior in college, Jim tragically lost both of his parents on the same day. Without warning, his parental "safety net" was gone. The emotional and financial support he knew would be there if needed vanished. For Jim, the loss of his parents was devastating.

As my health began to decline, the strain on our relationship began to take its toll. In September 1995, when I was hospitalized with PCP, it was obvious to me that my serious health condition was becoming increasingly difficult for Jim to handle. The possibility he might lose another loved one brought to mind the memories surrounding his parents' deaths. It was hard for Jim to come to the hospital. He frequently showed up an hour or so after he was expected, and when he finally arrived, he appeared to be nervous, fretful and rarely stayed long.

Shortly after my release from the hospital, my relationship with Jim changed. In my opinion, we both inwardly understood that the continuation of our relationship was not possible. At the time, I was convinced it was unlikely, if not impossible, for Jim to take on the role as my caretaker comfortably if or when my health failed, and I required constant care. I had no desire to burden Jim, someone I loved, with a task I felt he would not be able to manage well.

Since Jim and I owned our home together, we initially decided to continue to keep the house and live together as roommates. We were determined to stay friends and continued to do many things together, including attending a dinner club we had belonged to for several years. Every Wednesday night, a group of 20 friends would either meet at a restaurant or enjoy having dinner in one of the member's homes.

One Wednesday, in July of 1996, two of the women in our dinner club invited a guest, Chris Curry, to join the group for dinner. Chris enjoyed himself and soon became a regular member. Six months later, on January 1, 1997, Chris and I had lunch together. It was our first date.

On our second date, the two of us met for breakfast. I felt great when I got out of bed that morning and was excited about meeting Chris. Halfway through breakfast, I started to feel a little "funny" and by the time I had finished eating, I was slightly nauseous. We left the restaurant and within seconds I "lost" my breakfast in the parking lot. Chris, trying to be as helpful as possible, patiently waited while I finished throwing up.

I had no idea what was wrong. I was fine when I woke that morning, and in less than two hours, I felt as if I was about to die. My energy had evaporated and all I wanted to do was lie down, right in the parking lot. Chris, who lived nearby, insisted I come to his house.

When we arrived at Chris's place, I walked in the door and immediately headed to the sofa. He closed the blinds and took a seat in a chair across the room. I was not on the sofa long before I jumped up and made a dash for the nearby bathroom, arriving barely in time to lower my head into the toilet. A few minutes later, I was sitting on the toilet holding a trash can to catch the vomit. For the next three or four hours, I went back and forth from the sofa to the bathroom until finally, my stomach and intestines were empty.

The entire day, Chris sat in his darkened living room. He never turned on the television; he never read a book or magazine; he just sat quietly, checking occasionally to see if I needed anything. He sat in that chair for hours, doing nothing while I spent the entire day destroying his bathroom. With the exception of having PCP, I felt worse than I had at any other time in memory. Even more distressing, it was my second date with Chris. I remember thinking, *"it's not likely there will be a third."*

Late in the afternoon, Chris managed to get me in the car and drove me home. When we arrived, Jim was there and Chris insisted that the two of them take me to the hospital. Saint Luke's Hospital admitted me immediately; I had a fever of 105 degrees and was completely dehydrated. By the time I settled into a room, had blood drawn and an IV of fluids surging into my veins, it was after 11 p.m. Chris and Jim left, and I drifted off to sleep.

With the blinds in my hospital room closed, the room was mostly dark when I began to wake up the next day. I was groggy and had no idea if it was morning or afternoon. As my eyes grew accustomed to the dimly lit room, I noticed a figure sitting quietly in a chair. It was Chris. I said hello and asked, *"What time is it?"* He replied, *"It's about 11."* I followed up, *"How long have you been here?"* Chris said, *"Since about 8."* My heart fluttered and in that instant I fell in love.

Yes, Chris sat in the dark for three hours, waiting for me to wake up. He did this one morning after I threw up all over his house and turned his bathroom into a "hold your nose, enter at your own risk" zone. How could I not love this guy? More than 14 years later, I cannot imagine life without Chris. Perhaps "the messenger" sent him?

A year or so after Chris and I started dating, which had progressed to living together, we were having a discussion when the topic of the AIDS Quilt came up. We talked about the last time each of us had seen the Quilt. After I described my visit in the wheelchair, Chris, somewhat astonished said, *"I was there that day and remember seeing you, but **I never knew it was you**, until just now."*

Saying "goodbye" to Maggie

For 13 years, Maggie was an important part of my life. After Maggie was diagnosed with cancer that completely engulfed her kidneys and spleen, I made the painful decision to have her put to sleep. Like many animals, Maggie hated going to the vet. Dr. Goodman, Maggie's vet, compassionately agreed to make a house call so Maggie could take her last breath in the comfort of her own home.

The last two hours of her life, Maggie lay on the floor in our bedroom with her eyes wide open. Chris and I were also on the floor. The three of us spent those two hours staring at each other. At 3 p.m., Dr. Goodman and one of his vet techs, Jennifer, walked into the bedroom. Over the years, Jennifer had occasionally "moved in" with her dog, Peanut, to stay with Maggie whenever Chris and I were out of town.

As soon as Maggie saw Jennifer and Dr. Goodman arrive, she struggled to her feet and walked toward them slowly wagging her tail. I sat down cross-legged on the floor and Maggie immediately crawled into my lap. With Chris sitting on the floor beside me, we all watched patiently as Dr. Goodman used a pair of clippers to shave one of Maggie's front legs so he could easily locate a vein. The injection was painless. Maggie slowly lowered her head and with her nose resting on both our legs, peacefully took her last breath.

Today, on a shelf next to my bed, where I see it every morning, sits Maggie's urn containing her ashes, her collar, her favorite toy "hamburger," a picture of the two of us taken when I was skin and bones, weak and frail and she was a tiny puppy. The inscription on her urn reads, *"Maggie – You saved my life."*

Life was "dull" until September 2007

As soon as I recovered from PCP in the spring of 1996, I began a new HIV drug "cocktail," and my immune system improved. My CD4 count, which had been zero, slowly climbed into the low 200s, still dangerously low, but a marked improvement.

Between 1996 and 2007, my CD4 count hovered in the high 100s and low 200s. Other than struggling with one medical crisis after another, the most serious of which was an AIDS-related cancer, my life during those 12 years was much the same each day.

The HIV-related fatigue I had first experienced in 1995 continued to be a daily problem. I normally woke between 7 a.m. and 8 a.m., got up and felt OK until sometime after lunch. By the middle of the day, I was drained of energy. By 2 p.m. or 3 p.m., I was completely exhausted. I felt like an electrical appliance that had just been unplugged from the socket. Suddenly, I was too tired to concentrate, too tired to stay on my feet and even too tired to drive. As a result, I napped every afternoon until dinnertime, got up long enough to eat, watched TV for an hour or so and was back in bed by 9 p.m. Such was life for 12 years.

My social life sucked. All my friends knew that if they invited me to dinner, I had to be home and in bed by 9 p.m. When I was invited to a party or some other event lasting late into the night, I was the first to arrive, and the first to leave.

During those 12 years, my daily life was definitely routine – a dull routine. Even though I had limited energy, I spent a great deal of my "awake" time going from one school to another sharing my story. Each afternoon after I arrived home from a school, I collapsed and slept until dinner. All that changed in September 2007.

I am often asked why, after 30 years of having HIV, am I still living? It's a thought-provoking question, considering that more than 98 percent of those infected with this virus 30 years ago are no longer alive. How do I answer? Spiritually, I'm convinced "the messenger" and my decision to follow orders and share my story with others has had a significant role in prolonging my life. Hundreds of those who have heard my story agree.

"Dear Don ... The thing that impacted me the most was when you said the doctor told you and your friends that you only had two years to live and they all have passed except you. I think God is watching over you and as long as you keep on teaching kids he will keep you as healthy and safe as he can." – Stephanie

"Dear Mr. Carrel ... Before hearing you speak, I really wasn't concerned about HIV. I had an image of what teenage life would be like and that image included a lot of sexual interaction with a lot of different women. I would probably have never known the seriousness of HIV and AIDS if it had not been for your wise words.

I am sorry that you had to be infected with something so awful. I can't imagine how terrible it would be to wake up every morning knowing that someday you may have to go through everything that you've seen your friends go through. I never want to have that horrible burden.

That is why I thank God for giving you this disease, but keeping you alive, so that you may teach us what we need to know to stay alive and well. By coming and speaking to groups of kids, I guarantee that you save <u>many</u> lives, mine is probably one of them. Without your education on this topic, I wouldn't be nearly as safe, or nearly as smart as I am planning to be." – Alex

"Dear Don ... You are a heaven-sent inspiration and those who you've lost to this struggle are watching over you. I thank you for opening my eyes to a disease that affects millions and millions of people. May God bless you and keep you throughout your journey." – April

"Hey Don ... I admire you for taking the situation you are in and making the best of it. It's good that you use your experience to help others avoid the pain and life-changes you have endured. It must be great knowing you have the power to change somebody's life for the better. I thank God for saving your life this long after doctors thought you would only last a year or two. I will continue to pray for you and your cause." – Kevin

"Dear Don ... It is so awful that such an inspired person has such a horrible disease. But as we know, God won't give you more than you can handle and everything happens to certain people for certain reasons. I think this has happened to you so you can help others. I'm sure everyone appreciates what you're doing as much as me. Good luck with your project and may God be with you." – Whitney

Various factors allow some immune systems to survive longer than others. In my case, I apparently have a healthier than average immune system. I was rarely sick as a child and was extremely healthy as an adult until developing my first HIV-related illness 14 years after I was infected. I believe I was exposed to only one dose of HIV, on one occasion. The disease is known to progress more rapidly in those who have been infected multiple times. I've never smoked or abused drugs, both of which suppress the immune system. Throughout my life, I always have made an attempt to exercise and eat a fairly healthy diet, both of which help boost the immune system.

Earlier I talked about "defining" moments in our lives. In September 2007, I had such a moment. A couple of good friends, Paul and Rex, suggested I try a liquid nutritional supplement. The supplement contains vitamins, minerals, aloe, green tea and mangosteen, a fruit I had never heard of. After some research, I learned that mangosteen, which grows in abundance in most of Asia, is loaded with powerful antioxidants. Antioxidants are well known for their ability to boost immune system function.

At the time, I was taking a handful of six vitamins and minerals each morning and another six at night. I was taking two handfuls a day of what were supposedly the "best" vitamins and mineral supplements available. I've always believed that proper nutrition is vitally important to stay healthy and that it's impossible to get all the nutrients we need from our diets.

I had been choking down two handfuls of supplements for several years and while my health was not getting any better, it was at least holding its own. I readily agreed to stop swallowing 12 pills a day and replace them with two ounces of liquid nutrition.

Within two weeks of making the switch, I stopped taking naps. My energy levels returned to those I had not enjoyed since well before my bout with PCP in 1995. On the rare occasions I now nap, it's because it's a nice rainy afternoon and I want a nap, not because I need one.

Almost all my lab results have improved, including my CD4 count, which after remaining in the high 100s and low 200s for 12 years, now fluctuates between the mid-300s and high-400s. My AIDS-related cancer is in remission. Even though I "officially" have full-blown AIDS, I've not had a cold, the flu or any other illness that bears mentioning since I changed supplements nearly four years ago.

I have my life back. I get up at 6 a.m. or 7 a.m. and go to bed between 10 p.m. and 11 p.m. Socializing with friends is fun again and while I'm not an all-night party animal, I no longer have to be home and in bed by 9 p.m. When the occasion calls for it, I can be found on the dance floor, laughing and celebrating with friends – creating memories that will hopefully stay with me the next 12 years. I feel like a normal human being again.

While I have no scientific proof that the sudden turnaround in my energy and quality of life is due to my liquid nutritional supplement, I know of no other reason for the change.

I began sharing my story with others after "the messenger" in my dream instructed me to do so in 1995. After the first five years of my journey to help prevent HIV, I became increasingly frustrated. The more teenagers and adults who heard my story, the more I realized I was like one small fish in a huge ocean. There is a need for thousands of "me" traveling around the country, and the world, meeting with millions of youth to explain how HIV has a never-ending impact on life.

Ten years ago, I came up with the idea to put my story down on paper so it would hopefully reach many more people. I started writing and stopped many times. I stopped because I simply didn't have enough energy to accomplish the task.

I credit the liquid supplement I now take for the fact that my life has returned to "normal." My energy has improved, my attitude has improved and I have gone from simply surviving to thriving. I feel better than I have in 20 years. I'm convinced that without these changes in my life, you would not be reading this book, as I would not have had the strength to write it.

In the last three years, I've often wondered if "the messenger" had a role in giving me my life back. Perhaps "the messenger" knew I needed more energy before I could expand my audience to include you.

It might seem as if I'm interjecting a "commercial" for a supplement in my story. But I would be remiss if I failed to share this information with you. This book is about my life, and my life was transformed after I started this liquid nutritional supplement. Definitely a defining moment.

Further information is available at www.TrampleAIDS.com.

Call me "PJ"

During the 12 monotonous years between my recovery from PCP and the day I "got my life back" in 2007, one thrilling incident took place – an event I never thought I would be alive to experience. Maxwell Vincent Carrel was born. When Max was born on August 18, 2006, I became a grandfather!

My son, Chris, was only 11 when Dr. Wade told me I was HIV-positive and that I should expect to live only a few years. My primary focus during the early years of my infection was to stay alive long enough to see Chris and his brother, Matt, graduate from high school. Somehow, the possibility of ever being a grandfather never crossed my mind. It's as if my brain was reprogrammed and some-one erased the "grandfather" file. When I learned Chris and his wife, Jill, were expecting, I was in disbelief. Was I really going to live long enough to be a grandfather?

Hearing Jill was pregnant instantly brought back memories of my own childhood and the many hours I spent with my grandparents. When my dad's parents first became grandparents, they had no desire to be called "Grandma and Grandpa." They ended up as "Nanny and Poppy" while their six grandchildren were small. As the six of us became adults, Nanny and Poppy's names also made the transition to adulthood, and we started to call them "Nan and Pop."

Each one of Nan and Pop's grandchildren were adored, and the six of us often teased each other about who was their favorite. Nan and Pop had no favorite. Their love for each of us was endless. I may not have been the favorite grandchild, but I was the luckiest. I was privileged to be the only one of the six with Nan as she took her last breath at age 98. I was lucky enough to hold her hand, tenderly say my goodbyes and wipe away the last tear from her eye.

I have only wonderful memories of both Nan and Pop and I still miss them today. The same instant I heard I was going to be a grandfather, I named myself. To honor my grandfather's memory, I wanted to be "Poppy, Jr." – "PJ" for short. The name would not only constantly remind me of my relationship with Pop, it would prevent me from being "Grandpa Don." After all, I'm far too young to be called Grandpa!

The first time I held Max, an old fear resurfaced. Fear that I might die too soon. Later that evening, I sat quietly in his nursery with Jill's mother, Becky, as we watched our new grandson peacefully sleeping. Here are Becky's – aka – "Nana's" comments about that night:

I have known Don for a dozen years. When we first met, I called him Don. On August 18, 2006, he earned the lofty title "PJ" ... aka Poppy Junior ... for that was when our grandson, Maxwell Vincent Carrel was born. Max's arrival opened a whole new world for me as Nana, and also for PJ. We love that little guy more than life itself.

One evening, during a quiet time in Max's nursery, PJ and I sat together watching this newborn little boy sleep. It was an evening I will not forget. I do not remember who was sitting in the rocker or who was sitting on the floor. All I remember is that our hearts were open to talk about the life we both had in mind for this infant. Together, we shared our hopes and dreams of how Max would grow up with a happy childhood, excelling in school and becoming prosperous as an adult so he could carry the proud name of Maxwell Vincent...such a big name for such a little boy.

As most conversations begin, there is humor and the attempt to find a balance, sharing stories of our own children's birth. PJ and I started that way, too. But, soon, the talking turned serious. PJ confided a fear he had – that he would not live long enough for Max to remember him. He told his story about AIDS and how he fought this demon long enough to see his sons graduate from school.

In this quiet room, with the soft sounds of a baby sleeping, PJ asked a special favor of me. He asked that if anything should happen to him, would I, "Please make sure Max always remembers how much PJ loved him."

I promised PJ that his wishes would be carried out just as he asked. It was easy to do, because I feel the same way about Max.

After wiping our tears and sharing a hug, we quietly left the nursery and went downstairs where we found the rest of the family wiping away tears, as well. You see, what Don and I did not know was that the baby monitor from the nursery was broadcasting our entire conversation.

Don and I are now very blessed with a second grandchild, Kathryn Mae Carrel, born March 1, 2009. Let it be known that my promise to PJ will be carried out for Katie, Max's little sister, just as it will for Max.

I am so thankful that Grandchildren and Grandparents are a wonderful part of God's plan. – Nana aka Becky Mackey

As Nana mentioned, I not only have a grandson, Max, I also have been blessed with a granddaughter, Katie, who turned two in March 2011. Katie's "big brother," Max, starts kindergarten this fall. Both Max and Katie love spending time with "PJ" and "Grandpa Chris." Yes, my partner, who is actually 11 years younger than me, has been tagged as "Grandpa Chris." PJ and Grandpa Chris plan to be alive and well for many more years. Who knows? Maybe "the messenger" plans for me to be a great-grandparent.

CHAPTER 7

"It's all in the family"

One of the first things I did once I made the decision to write this book was to drag out the many boxes of the letters I've received over the past 15 years from high-school students who have heard my story. As I re-read thousands of letters, I noticed many of the writers made reference to something I failed to include during my presentations. I provided little insight into my personal struggle with HIV/AIDS and even less into how having HIV and AIDS has impacted my family and friends.

Dear Don … I thought maybe instead of telling us so much about your friends that had the disease you should have told us more about yourself." – Maggie

"Dear Don … The thing that had the biggest impact on me was when you told us about your friends and how you had to watch them suffer. That is horrible and I'm really sorry … One thing I wanted to know more about was how did your family react and was it hard to tell them?" – Amanda

"Dear Don Carrel … Your speech was very effective and got the point across. However, you might want to try talking more about yourself and how this has affected your family members and your personal relationship with them. It might be hard for you to do and that's understandable, but it might help you to become a stronger person inside. … You have taught us the importance of life and have helped save hundreds of lives." – Melissa

Originally, I had no plans to include nearly as many details about my personal struggle with HIV in this book. I changed my mind after reading hundreds, if not thousands, of letters expressing the same sentiments as those quoted above. Including the thoughts of my family and closest friends only made sense once I realized that their reaction to my HIV status is part of my story.

Several months ago, I emailed a brief message to my closest family members and friends asking them to send me *"a few thoughts about how you felt when you learned I was HIV-positive and how my having HIV has impacted your life and your attitude about HIV."* In the previous chapter, I included comments from my parents, my sons, my sister, Debbie, my sister-in-law, Anita, and a few of my closest friends.

This chapter is comprised of the responses I received from other members of my family and a few close friends. Before I share their comments, I would like you to know that the reaction of all my family and close friends upon learning I was infected with HIV has been nothing but loving and supportive. During my 15-year journey to prevent others from contracting HIV, I've met a number of teens and young adults who have not had the family support and acceptance that I've received from my loved ones. Personally, I've talked with a handful of high school and college students who were literally "kicked out of the house" after their parents discovered they had HIV. My heart aches for those with HIV/AIDS who are homeless, simply because they're not as fortunate as I have been.

My brother, Dave

Dave, my brother, is 20 months younger than my younger sister, Debbie. When we were kids Debbie was very protective of her "baby brother," especially whenever I had an issue with my annoying "little brother." After high school, Dave chose to work in the family business and did not follow Debbie and me to K-State. Since we were separated by distance, Dave and I did not see each other often and our visits normally consisted of a few hours together. As a result, early in my adult life, I developed a closer bond with Debbie than I did with Dave.

In the late 1970s when I "came out of the closet," Dave was not comfortable having a gay brother. His job required him to spend much of his time with blue-collar workers, who found nothing wrong with telling "gay" jokes or making derogatory comments about gays. Personally, Dave did not have a problem accepting my sexual orientation, but he found it rather embarrassing to discuss the fact I was gay with most of his acquaintances.

After I closed *Kitchens Plus* and moved back to Kansas City, I told Dave about my HIV status. His reaction was immediate. It was almost as if someone "flipped a switch." The fact that I was gay was suddenly no longer an issue. For Dave, having a gay brother paled in comparison to having one with HIV, an illness that could rob him of his brother at any time.

Since the day Dave first learned of my HIV status, my relationship with him has done nothing but grow closer. My partner, Chris, and I frequently go out and enjoy margaritas and Mexican food with Dave and his wife, Anita. On many occasions, other friends, both gay and straight, join the four of us. My health status and the nature of my relationship with Chris is no longer a "secret" and is common knowledge among Dave's friends. In the last 20 years of my adult life, I've been able to spend more time with my brother than with my sister. I'm now thrilled to have a close relationship with both of my siblings.

When I asked Dave if I could share the story about how his attitude took an immediate "about face" once he learned of my HIV status, he readily gave his consent. However, he did say, ***"But give me a break. My initial attitude about you being gay was one I held in the 1970s. That was a long time ago, and times have changed. I would not have felt the same way today."***

Dave's sudden acceptance of my sexual orientation after learning I had HIV reminds me, in some ways, of the reaction that Jill, my daughter-in-law, had a number of years ago when she first discovered I was gay and HIV-positive. My son, Chris, revealed both bits of information during the same conversation a couple of months after the two of them started dating.

Jill sent me a letter. At the time she wrote this letter, she was 22 and had known Chris, who was then 24, for three years. I would like to share a portion of Jill's letter with you.

<u>My daughter-in-law, Jill</u>

Dear Don,

Chris did not talk about you very much when we first started dating. We began dating in March, and it was late

August before he told me the whole story. One day, Chris noticed I had a red ribbon pinned on my backpack and asked why I had it there. I told him I couldn't even remember where or when I got the ribbon. He seemed intrigued, but dropped the subject.

A couple of weeks later, he asked again about my red ribbon. Before I could even answer he said, "My dad has AIDS." And he started to cry. In the three years I had known Chris, it's the only time I had ever seen him cry.

Until then, I had never known anyone with AIDS, or even anyone who was personally affected by the disease. After we talked about your health for a little while, he said you were gay. By that time, I was kind of numb and the fact you were gay didn't even affect me. So that's kind of how it was, first you had AIDS and then you were gay.

I don't really have any specific thoughts about your lifestyle. I'm just worried about your health.

I guess I feel that if we were all the same, things would be very boring. Since we're gay and straight, white and black, happy and sad, smart and not so smart, this world we live in is a great place. Of course at times, there are some judgmental folks, but to hell with them, right? – Love, Jill

My daughter-in-law, Audie

My youngest son, Matt, is a talented, successful tattoo artist in Indianapolis. He and his wife, Audie, live on a few acres along with their four "babies" – all of which are large, loved and slightly spoiled dogs. Audie and Matt haven't known each other nearly as long as Chris and Jill, and Audie learned about my HIV status years after most of my family members. Here are Audie's comments:

Not long after Matt and I started dating, Matt told me you were gay and HIV-positive. To be perfectly honest, I didn't have much of a reaction. Over the years, I have had several friends, both straight and gay, who have been HIV-positive and some have passed.

However, I was shocked when Matt told me you had been positive since the early 1980s. Ryan White, who was from Indiana where I lived, was the first person I ever heard of that had HIV/AIDS. At that time, I remember no one was surviving and there was no successful treatment.

My "California Cousins"

While growing up, my sister, brother and I spent many hours hanging out with our three cousins, who now all live in Northern California. All six of us are within five years of age, and our relationships have always been more like that of siblings than of cousins. When I talk about my treatment history in Chapter 12, you'll read the "mini-pad" story written by my cousin, Pam. Following are comments from my other two cousins, Katy (KT) and Bill, and Bill's wife, Gwenly.

My cousin, KT

There were six of us cousins who grew up together in the Midwest. We spent summer vacations and holidays together; we were as close as siblings and still have a strong sense of family.

I remember the phone call from my dear cousin so many years ago. Don called from Kansas City to California to tell me he had HIV. I had recently come out and was living in San Francisco and understood the seriousness of Don's call.

In the late 1980s gay men were dying in frightening numbers. It seemed fairly certain to me that death was near for Don. There was no cure or medication that worked. It still makes me extremely sad to think of Don not being around. It also makes me very angry to hear what drug companies charge, and how insurance companies have treated HIV patients like Don.

I remember thinking that my favorite cousin Don was going to die and there wasn't anything I could do to help. I was devastated. How could that happen in our family? How could it happen to Cousin Don?

I still get very sad when I think of Don getting sick, but more than sad I remain in awe and respect of Don's tenacity in beating this awful disease. He's had some tough moments, but hasn't given up. I am incredibly proud of all Don has accomplished since finding out he has HIV, realizing his dream and accomplishing his 'mission' in this lifetime.

He has touched many thousands of lives and has undoubtedly saved many of them. Don's life has changed, and so has the life of everyone who knows him. I am so proud of – and love – my cousin, Don.

My cousin, Bill

I wasn't as much shocked, as I was saddened when I learned that my cousin, Don, had been diagnosed with HIV. Don has always been an outgoing, sociable guy, and I knew he was active in the gay community, so I it didn't come as a shock that he became infected. But knowing that AIDS is often fatal, I didn't think Don would be alive that much longer, and it made me sad to think about the challenges he'd be facing in everyday life.

Don has been crusading tirelessly over the years, spreading the word about AIDS prevention to high-school groups and others. I'm proud of my Cousin Don and admire his perseverance. He's touched many lives, including my own, about thoughts and awareness of AIDS and HIV.

Gwenly, Cousin Bill's wife

Our children began to know Cousin Don, when he was making frequent trips to San Francisco for treatments with a specialist. Before that time, Nick and Marika had only met him when they were very young children at a couple of family reunions. They never really knew that he was living with AIDS.

When he started coming to San Francisco so often, we would get together for family dinners with Don, his partner Chris, and the other cousins who live in the Bay Area. It was not a secret as to why he was visiting so frequently. When we explained to our then nine-year-old daughter and 13-year-old son that Cousin Don was living with AIDS, there weren't many questions. The most poignant of them was, "How long will he live?" Almost nine years later, our daughter, Marika, won the grand prize in an HIV/AIDS Art Awareness campaign. Her winning work is of a girl with AIDS; she is crying and wrapping a red ribbon around her body.

When questioned by a reporter about where she got the inspiration for her beautiful piece, Marika replied, "I am in Art 2 … and for our last assignment we were required to enter a piece for the AIDS competition, or create a piece about another controversial issue. When I was given the choice, I knew right away that I would enter the AIDS competition because my dad's cousin has had AIDS for about 20 years."

Please Note: If you would like to see Marika Carrel's award winning piece of art entitled *"Don't Turn Your Back on AIDS"* you can do so by going to the following website: http://www.lamorindaweekly.com/archive/issue0322/Dont-Turn-Your-Back-on-AIDS.html.

My aunt and uncle, Marilyn & Bob
Pam, Bill and KT's parents

As your aunt and uncle, we wondered why you were in such a hurry to get married when you graduated from college. We think back then we were aware of your possible lifestyle. And when you did get HIV/AIDS, we were sad for you and your mother who took it so hard. We accepted and loved you and Katy from the time we knew you were gay, even though at times we didn't understand why you chose that very difficult route to live.

We also want to speak for Nanny (Don's grandmother) *who was a woman before her time. She would fight tigers to uphold your right to be who you were and she loved you very much. We believe being genetically predisposed to be homosexual, it was not a total surprise – you didn't choose the lifestyle – it chose you. We hope, Don, this is what you wanted. Good luck on your book, and we do want an autographed copy after it is published.*

My brother-in-law,
COL Scott King, U.S. Army

I have known Don for nearly 20 years. I grew up in the South and had a very conservative upbringing. My parents raised me in a Christian home, and I attended a private Southern Baptist Church School in Atlanta. Most of my teachers were graduates of Bob Jones University or Tennessee Temple, some of the most conservative schools in America. I came to know Jesus Christ as my personal savior when I was in first grade.

After high school, I attended West Point. In one of my classes, we had an in-depth study of HIV/AIDS focusing on the U.S. Policy regarding the disease. This was the first time that I fully examined the disease and how it was transmitted from individual to individual.

I participated in Desert Storm and upon my return attended a wedding where I met a beautiful lady, Debbie, Don's sister. I immediately fell in love and after months of pursuing, Debbie finally agreed to marry me. While we were dating, Don was living in the same town and was the first person in Debbie's family that I met. Debbie told me about Don's sexual orientation and his HIV virus. This was the first time I knowingly had socialized with someone who was gay and had HIV. I had heard some of the public discussions that AIDS was GOD's punishment for homosexuals.

How was I going to act? Debbie has a very close relationship with Don. She followed him to college and even lived in some of the same houses that he had. Don was also close to Debbie's three kids and always gave them the best birthday presents. I thought about my relationship with my own sister. There is nothing that would ever come between my sister and me. I realized that Debbie and Don had a similar relationship. I also saw the relationship that Don had with Debbie's kids and realized that is the same type of relationship that I was trying to have with my sister's boys.

I realized that though I personally did not fully understand Don's sexual orientation, I did understand Don and his actions toward Debbie and the kids. I decided that I would go into a relationship with Don with open arms and the rest has been a great history.

I have had the opportunity to travel much of the world and met some great people in my career in the Army, but I don't think I have met anyone like Don Carrel. Don has a very resilient strength as demonstrated by the numerous times he has been hospitalized. I don't know anyone that pursues life with the passion in all things that he does.

I am thankful for my relationship with Don and the relationship he has with our children. I believe I laugh the hardest when I am in his presence. I admire him for what he's done with his life by talking to youth about HIV and AIDS. Don Carrel has taught me much about life and how to live it to the fullest. I'm glad to have him as my Brother-in-Law and as my friend! – Scott King

My nieces and nephews

My brother, Dave, has two children, Jon and Michelle. My sister, Debbie, has four children, Aaron, Laura and Andrea from her first marriage and Ryan from her current marriage to Scott. Here are the comments I received from all six of my nieces and nephews and those of Aaron's wife, Krista.

My nephew, Aaron – Age 31

I first found out that you had HIV in 1994 or 1995 when I was a freshman or sophomore in high school. At that point in my life, I knew you were gay, but the HIV diagnosis added a whole new "element," especially after I learned you had HIV for over a decade by the time I found out.

I remember thinking "Well, if he's had it for a long time and everybody has been around him, why should I worry now?" That being said, I think it probably made me overly cautious at first. Even though in high school we had HIV/AIDS prevention classes, I still found myself washing my hands more often when I was at your house, when you cooked dinner, etc. I remember one incident shortly after I found out when Mom kissed you on the lips. I thought to myself, why would she do that now that she knows he's HIV-positive? Even though I knew it wasn't transferrable that way, I still couldn't help but thinking, why risk it?

As I grew more comfortable in my own right, I still refrained from telling anyone that I had a gay uncle, let alone one with HIV. I lived in rural Kentucky then and everyone was very con-servative and being gay or having HIV was not something that anybody had any reference point for. No one ever talked about knowing anyone gay, and especially gay and HIV-positive.

Even in college, where everybody is supposed to have an "open mind," I still didn't talk about it. Krista was probably the first person I ever told. After I told her, and as it became more acceptable, I slowly started talking about it with people as the issue arose.

Today I don't typically think twice about it and the fear I had about being around you has worn off over the years. It's like Krista's comment about the boogey man, most things are not as nearly as scary as they may first seem.

I know Krista and I, Mom, the girls, and everybody else is proud of what you have done for HIV/AIDS awareness and pre-vention. And that is what I typically follow up with when I talk to anyone about having an uncle who is HIV-positive. I tell them about all of the good things you do now.

Krista, Aaron's wife – Age 31

Aaron, I remember the night you told me your uncle had HIV. We were at Grandma Shirley's house and I was going to meet Don the next day. Initially I was very scared. The only real exposure I had ever had to HIV/AIDS were the movies, "And the Band Played On" and "Philadelphia." I remember thinking how awful the disease was because if you get it, there is no cure.

In one of the movies they showcased all of these famous people who had died from HIV/AIDS at the end. I was scared at first because I never met anyone who had HIV. I didn't know very much about the disease. I remember hearing a little about it in school growing up and they talked about the different ways you could/couldn't get HIV/AIDS. I think I was afraid of the unknown and seeing how the disease was depicted in the movies.

Uncle Don was my first real lesson in learning that just because you have the disease, it's not a death sentence. Here's this guy, larger than life, who if you didn't know he had AIDS, you would never guess it. He is out educating others and living a healthy, normal life.

Over the years, I've gotten to know Don as a person and as an uncle and now it is easy to forget he has AIDS. AIDS is like the Boogeyman in the closet. You initially have all this fear of the unknown until you turn on the light and see that there was never anything in the closet to be afraid of in the first place.

My niece, Laura – Age 26

I remember sitting in the auditorium that day looking over my shoulder and staring at my mother standing in the back of the room with my sister, Andrea, by her side. They were staring at the other students pouring in from all the classes and promptly taking their seats. I went to school here, but my sister did not. My mom took Andrea out of school so she could attend the speech my uncle was about to give.

HIV/AIDS is a surreal thing to a teenager. A teenager doesn't often think of his or her own mortality. In its place are thoughts of indestructibility and prowess. They are content to turn a blind eye to the real threat of the growing number of teenagers infected by HIV.

This is why my uncle has come today. He has lived most of his adult life with HIV and planned to tell my classmates about the dangers of unprotected sex. Through personal experiences and stories, he proudly told my peers what his life is like on a daily basis. He told us about the numerous medications he takes daily and how much they cost each day. I remember a gasp going through the auditorium when my uncle told us how much he pays for his medications. It was startling.

All those numbers. I told myself that day that I wasn't going to be another number. Another statistic. Another lost face. I have secretly thought my uncle was brave for telling others of his disease so that he may save just one other person from the experiences he has had to endure. Looking around the auditorium, I saw an array of expressions on the faces of my classmates: sympathy, shock, fear, boredom, but none was more beautiful than that of my uncle's. An expression of determination filled his face. Determination, so the people sitting around me would make smart choices regarding sex. Determination so my generation would be the last to be plagued by the pandemic virus.

"The difference between impossible and possible lies in a person's determination" ~ Tommy Lasorda. That is the lesson my uncle had to share. Determination makes all the difference. It is that difference that my classmates and I took away that day as we somberly made our way back to class. We were all a little more determined to not be another number.

My niece, "Andie" - Age 25

I can remember being a little girl, around the age of six or seven, and about to take a drink of my Uncle Don's water when he quickly took it from me and said, "No, no, no sweetheart, that's mine." This was during the period of time where doctors were unsure of exactly how HIV was spread and some thought it could be transmitted through saliva.

Years passed and scientists learned the virus is passed from sharing needles or sexually transmitted by someone who has HIV, not by drinking out of someone's glass.

My Uncle has defied death and is a living miracle. He explains the danger of unsafe sex to students of all ages. He is not just another STD video shown in health class; he lives with the disease every day. He knows the harsh reality of what having HIV can do to your life. I believe that even after he is gone, his story will still be told and will save lives.

You are one of the strongest people I know. You have made me a better person in more ways than you can imagine. Uncle Don, I love you and I am so proud to be your niece.

My nephew, Ryan – Age 17

Uncle Don, I know this isn't exactly what you were looking for, but I'm not sure that I'm really informed enough to be giving a good opinion about HIV, so I just tried to do what I could.

When I first learned that you were gay, I was young. I saw how you and Chris loved each other, so I didn't see this as being a big deal. As I have grown up, I've witnessed other people's opinions about gay people. I believe gay people are just like everyone else and I never feel uncomfortable or awkward when I'm around you and Chris.

It has helped me understand many of my peers who are gay and I stick up for them, as high school can be a hard time for many homosexuals to feel accepted. I have always felt blessed for having you as an uncle and you have taught me many things directly and indirectly. With what I've learned, I believe I can be a better and more understanding person when I encounter people with differences than my own.

My nephew, Jon – Age 26

Thanks to my Uncle Don, I have learned a lot about HIV over the course of my life. Many people, especially teens and young adults, have an "out of sight, out of mind" mindset when it comes to this disease.

I am fortunate to have an uncle who takes AIDS awareness to the next level. Between his involvement in the AIDS walk and other activities like speaking to countless number of teens, my Uncle Don has helped make a huge impact on many lives including mine. He has greatly affected my life in a positive way.

With all that I have learned, I have definitely become aware of the disease and how to prevent it. Living safely when it comes to preventing this disease is a simple task and an easy message to learn as long as people are willing to listen.

My niece, Michelle – Age 22

By the time I was old enough to even know what AIDS, the four-letter acronym was, I still didn't know much about it. All I knew was that it was a very serious disease, and my Uncle was infected with it. I remember being told that those afflicted don't have a very long life expectancy. I can recall the initial shock of it. Grasping that my Uncle Don could pass away any time and there was nothing I, or anyone else, could do about it.

Whenever I think about it, if I were in his shoes, I would focus on enjoying what time I had left. Yet, nonetheless, he focuses on educating others rather than himself. He's dedicated to the pre-vention of HIV in the young adults of America. Personally, I don't think I could ever muster the willpower to go up on a stage and tell such personal aspects of my life to complete strangers.

Since the first time I heard him speak about his life with the dis-ease, I have seen my uncle as an inspiration. A symbol saying, "Yes, life can seem hopeless sometimes, but you just have to grit your teeth, get up and try to make the best of what you were given."

More from my "Family"

My "family" not only includes my relatives, it includes my closest friends. I'm ending this chapter with comments from five of my favorite "family" members. Damon, Dottie, Kathy, Jennifer and CP have all been my friends for many years.

Damon Roberts, my first partner

Dear Don,

Devastated — it was the first thought that came to mind in my reaction to the news of your HIV-positive status. Even though our relationship had ended in the early eighties, another relationship of friendship had begun. Love should never stop; rather it should morph over time.

Another reaction was more personal — "Could I be HIV-positive, too?" Going to the Free Health Clinic for my HIV test in the mid-eighties certainly gave me a platform to inventory my entire life. Thankfully, I'm not infected. How I came through that time of my life unscathed is a blessing.

Looking back to the nineties, I thought it odd that your family was throwing you a major 45th birthday party, but seeing you in that wheelchair as a ghost of the person I knew, defined it all in a split second. You simply weren't going to be around for another birthday party. It was a little too much to take, knowing the event was probably the last time I would see you alive. The drive home was torture, almost as torturous as trying to paint on a "birthday party face" in your presence.

As your grandmother Nanny often said, "Oh, he's a special one, you know!" Over and over again, you have proven that voice correct, especially in what I consider the second life given to you. I would like to think that Nan is up there beaming at all the good you have accomplished, for the metropolitan area's youth and the life-saving information you have conveyed in countless venues and schools.

I'm still shaking my head every time I see you, Don Carrel, knowing the journey you have endured and the experiences that have brought you to this day. I am so proud of you, wishing both Chris and you continued happiness together. Keep passionate for what needs to be done!

Oh, by the way...Nanny was absolutely right...I knew it then, I have witnessed it since!

With best wishes, in the love of friendship
— Damon

Dottie Smith, my friend for nearly 30 years

I first met Dottie in 1982, before I opened *Kitchens Plus*. Dottie is a sales representative and is the first person I ordered merchandise from prior to opening my store. In fact, at the time of our first appointment, I had not yet picked a location for my business. For our first meeting, Dottie met me at my home and we worked at the kitchen table.

I remember the day I received a call from Don asking if I would meet him at his store. I am a sales rep and he and was a very special customer of mine. As I sat in his office, he told me that he was HIV-positive.

I remember not knowing what to say. In our business, at the time, I had several friends who had contracted HIV, and only one was still alive and he was gravely ill.

Don told me that he was taking medication and was going to do anything in his power to beat this. I have never known anyone to take the offense in his or her illness battle like Don did.

Kathy Michaels, my friend for 25 years

Kathy Michaels was one my valued employees who worked at *Kitchens Plus* until the day I closed the store. She was there the same time as Jo and LeAnne. At the time I hired Kathy, she was a single parent raising a small son on her own.

I remember when I first heard about the AIDS Quilt with panels of people that had passed from AIDS. Before that, I didn't even know that HIV/AIDS existed. Even though I had an uncle who died from AIDS, I learned so much about HIV through you.

I also remember once when I told you I was going on a date, you tried to give me condoms, just in case I might need one. When I think back to that episode, I smile (You were my big brother). – Kathy Michaels

Jennifer Moore, my friend for nearly 30 years

I first met Jen when *Kids Plus Me* opened in 1993. At the time, Jen had two young daughters, Allison and Emily, who loved to shop for toys. Jen and her girls were in my store weekly to either shop for themselves or for a birthday present for a friend of one of the girls. In addition to being regular shoppers we became good friends. Years after we first met, Allison and Emily had the opportunity to hear my story while they were attending high school.

Hi Don ... You wanted my thoughts about how I felt when you told me you were HIV-positive. I remember feeling devastated; I had no idea how long I would have you in my life. My girls were young at the time and emotionally attached to you. I didn't want them to lose you because you're one of their positive male role models. I didn't want you to have to suffer and worried the first year that I would get a phone call and you would be in the hospital with the end near.

Thankfully you have been proactive about your disease and you have thrived, so I no longer worry about losing you daily. The girls and I feel so lucky to have you and Chris in our lives. You have both been so supportive through the years.

I have become aware of AIDS issues that I would have been less concerned about without knowing you. I'm proud of you for educating teenagers; you ARE saving lives. The kids relate to you because many of them don't have another adult who will talk to them honestly about sex. I remember one of the AIDS walks where a huge crowd of teenagers came to walk with you because they liked you. Kids brag about being your friend, you have rock star status! Your book will do a lot of good. It's the next part of your mission. – Love, Jen

CP Ward, my friend for nearly 40 years

Last but not least are comments from CP. I met CP nearly 40 years ago – shortly after Karen and I were married. CP was once my hair stylist and frequently shopped at *Kitchens Plus* and ate lunch in *The Croissant Café*. After I closed my businesses in Manhattan, CP occasionally made trips to Kansas City and, when in town, she always stopped at *Kids Plus Me* to visit. The last time she came to my toy store was in 1995, just before I was hospitalized with PCP.

Don has been a friend and important part of my life for nearly 40 years. Years ago, when we both lived in Manhattan, he was a "friend in-deed" as I went through a difficult transition in my life.

After he moved to Kansas City, I went to visit him at his new store, Kids Plus. His health and physical appearance were deteriorating and in 1995, it became apparent that death was imminent.

I felt so helpless – a feeling that evolved into sorrow and settled permanently into a corner of my heart when I heard – the false rumor – that Don died in 1996.

Then one day last year, (2010) Don unexpectedly walked into my workplace in Manhattan and asked to see me. After the inevitable "Oh my God, I thought you were dead," and "What happened, you don't look like you have ever been sick a day in your life," I realized a miracle had occurred that brought about our reconnection.

But, as I heard his story of the past 15 years, I realized the real miracle of Don's life has been his mission to connect with thousands of teens and share his message. For that, we are all blessed. – CP Ward

I'll never forget that summer day in 2010, when I literally "stumbled" upon CP's salon while visiting my old stomping grounds in Manhattan. By chance, I happened to be in a wellness office filled with massage therapists, chiropractors and nutritional specialists. On the counter were business cards for everyone working there. As I stopped to pick up someone's card, I noticed one for "CP Ward – Stylist" I had not seen or spoken to CP in 15 years, and the thought of reconnecting with her was thrilling.

I asked if CP happened to be working that day. She was downstairs having lunch. One of the staff members went down to tell her she had an "out-of-town" visitor. She came up stairs, looked at me and just stared. I could see the "wheels turning" as she attempted to figure who her out-of-town visitor happened to be. Even though we had been friends for many years, she did not know me until I said, *"Hi, CP,"* after which, she recognized my voice. Initially, she thought I was a ghost. I looked nothing like the sickly, frail friend she had last seen 15 years earlier. In fact, she thought I was dead.

Back to the "Presentation"

Well, I definitely interrupted the flow of my typical HIV presentation. I've revealed a great deal of information about my personal struggle and how being HIV-positive affected my family and friends. However, I've barely touched on my physical struggle with HIV, which will be discussed in Chapter 12 about the treatment of HIV.

My "presentation" picks up again starting with the next chapter, the "History of HIV/AIDS."

CHAPTER 8

History of HIV/AIDS

I started reading everything I could find about HIV/AIDS more than 25 years ago. My interest in learning about the "new disease" that appeared to be infecting gay men started during the earliest days of the epidemic and increased once I started to suspect I could be HIV-positive. My desire to know everything about AIDS intensified once I learned that in fact, I was infected with what was considered a fatal disease.

When I began to share my story in an attempt to help prevent HIV, one of my priorities was always to provide accurate information. However, determining what is accurate information can be difficult to do for several reasons. First, those individuals and organizations that provide information on HIV history, statistics, prevention, etc. often have differences of opinion. For example, according to a number of sources, an estimated 1.2 million Americans are currently HIV-positive. However, I've seen projections that the number of infected Americans living with HIV is closer to 2 million. Second, one must realize that HIV/AIDS statistics are always changing. What is important is that you get an understanding of how the disease is trending.

In this book I'm making every effort to provide you with accurate, up-to-date information. All the following historical and statistical facts and figures were gathered from what I consider to be very reliable sources. In addition, most of the statistical information in this book was included only after identical information appeared in two or more sources.

The sources include: the Centers for Disease Control (CDC); the UNAIDS latest Global Summary of the AIDS Epidemic; the World Health Organization (WHO); WebMD; Wikipedia; Avert.org (Avert is an international HIV and AIDS charity, based in the UK, working to avert HIV and AIDS worldwide, through education, treatment and care.); the Kaiser Family Foundation (www.kff.org/hivaids/timeline/hivtimeline.cfm); AIDS.about.com; UNFPA.org/aids and www.infoplease.com/spot/aidstimeline2.html.

I cannot discuss the history of HIV/AIDS without putting in a plug for my favorite book on the subject. My desire to learn more about the history of this epidemic led me to read the book, **And the Band Played On: Politics, People and the AIDS Epidemic** authored by Randy Shilts and published in 1987. This book was extensively researched and is a fascinating account of the discovery and spread of HIV/AIDS during the early years of the epidemic. Shilts' book begins by discussing events that occurred in 1976, just prior to the time of the earliest suspicions that there might be a "new disease" having the potential to kill millions. The book is written in chronological order and describes in detail the early days of the epidemic up to May 1987.

Shilts' book was compelling for me, partially because it discusses what was going on in Africa, Western Europe (primarily in Paris) and the United States during the same time period. It clearly illustrates how researchers around the world were able to piece together information to begin the fight against AIDS. Sadly, the book also points out the political climate that helped contribute to the U.S. government's indifference to what was initially perceived as a disease that only impacted gay men.

In 1993, **And the Band Played On** was made into an HBO film starring many big-screen actors including Richard Gere, Lily Tomlin, Matthew Modine, Steve Martin, Alan Alda, among others. The film, the book and the author all received many awards including a Pulitzer Prize for Shilts. If you are interested in learning more about the beginning of the AIDS pandemic, I highly recommend you check out this book.

Tragically, Randy Shilts developed PCP in 1992, Kaposi's sarcoma (an AIDS related cancer) in 1993 and died from complications of AIDS in 1994. Despite the fact Shilts was dying and on oxygen, he managed to attend the Los Angeles screening of HBO's **And the Band Played On** in August 1993, six months before his death.

Randy Shilts' book helped me understand in detail how the AIDS epidemic actually began and how the disease managed to become a worldwide pandemic. I'm often asked how HIV/AIDS got started and how things have changed since the beginning of the disease. The following HIV/AIDS timeline is a "Cliff notes" version of the history of HIV/AIDS.

Prior to 1970

HIV, the virus that causes AIDS, more than likely transferred from monkeys to humans living in Africa sometime between 1880 and 1920. It has been known for a number of years that certain viruses can pass from one species to another. When a virus transfers from animals to humans, it is known as zoonosis.

While it is possible that people were dying from AIDS before 1900, the first documented case was a man who died in the Congo in 1959. Plasma samples that were taken before his death in 1959 were retained for research purposes and when tested years later, it was discovered these samples contained traces of HIV.

Some chimpanzees have a simian immunodeficiency virus (SIV) that, when transmitted to humans, results in HIV infection. On a number of occasions, a teenager has asked me, sometimes in jest and sometimes in all seriousness, *"Did humans first get HIV because someone had sex with a monkey?"* The question always results in a group of laughing, giggling or red-face teens. Since the most common method of transmission of the virus between humans involves sex, I can easily understand why many teenagers, and even some adults, have posed this question.

The most commonly accepted theory of how HIV was transferred from monkeys to humans is the "hunter theory." For hundreds of years, monkeys have been a source of food and their hides a source of clothing for natives living in the jungles of Africa. HIV was more than likely transferred to humans as a result of chimps/monkeys being killed and eaten or their blood getting into cuts or wounds on the hunter. In other words, HIV probably found its way into mankind through the butchering and consumption of monkey meat.

Given the evidence we have, it is apparent that Africa is the continent where the transfer of HIV to humans first occurred. Monkeys from Asia and South America do not have SIV that causes HIV in humans. In addition, approximately 33 million people worldwide have HIV, and 22 million of them are Africans. Since 67 percent of those infected with HIV/AIDS worldwide are Africans, it easily leads me to conclude this pandemic started there.

A number of theories attempt to explain why the epidemic grew so rapidly in Africa in its early days. One of the theories involves testing for an oral polio vaccine that was given to nearly a million people in Sub-Saharan Africa in the late 1950s. To reproduce the live polio vaccine, it needed to be cultivated in living tissue. Some believe the polio vaccine given to Africans in the 1950s was cultivated in kidney cells taken from local chimps infected with SIV. This theory would explain why a large number of people in Africa subsequently became infected with HIV.

Another possible theory involves the use of contaminated needles during the same period. In the 1950s, the use of disposable plastic syringes was common and seen as a cheap, sterile way to administer medicines. However, to healthcare professionals working on inoculation and other medical programs in the poorer regions of Africa, the huge number of syringes needed would have been cost prohibitive. It's likely that one single syringe would have been used to inject multiple patients. This would easily have transferred any viral particles from one person to another.

In the 1970s

HIV probably first entered the U.S. and parts of Western Europe sometime between the late 1960s and the early to mid-1970s. During the decade of the 1970s, the pandemic gathered steam as the yet-to-be-discovered virus began spreading throughout the world completely unnoticed. In hindsight, it is likely that a female Danish physician died of the disease in 1977 after being infected while working at a medical clinic in Africa. In 1978, at least three women in Paris lost their lives from the same disease. These European women died several years before the first deaths from the disease occurred in the United States.

1980

In 1980, four Americans died of what would later be called AIDS. All four of those known to have died from this "new disease" that year were gay or bisexual men.

1981

This was the year I believe I was infected with HIV, three years before the virus was actually discovered, and four years before there was a test available to determine if someone was HIV-positive.

Starting in 1981, the CDC noticed an alarming rate of a rare cancer, called Kaposi's sarcoma (KS), appearing in otherwise healthy gay and bisexual men. This form of cancer can cause multiple tumors in the lymph nodes and/or lesions on the skin that are reddish/purple in color.

Prior to 1981, KS was normally a benign form of cancer that occurred primarily in elderly men. However, the KS affecting these younger men who had sex with men (MSM) was far more aggressive than the typical cases of KS in elderly men and often resulted in death. Since the initial individuals diagnosed with KS in 1981 were all MSM, the CDC first referred to this new disease as "gay cancer."

About the same time the medical community and the CDC started to notice KS in gay and bisexual men, a few medical professionals in both California and New York also started to treat a number of MSM for a rare lung infection, Pneumocystis carinii pneumonia (PCP).

Once the CDC discovered that the men with PCP, as well as the men suffering from KS, had compromised immune systems, the term "gay cancer" became obsolete and the disease was renamed GRID – Gay Related Immune Deficiency. The name GRID could be applied to MSM who were suffering from either or both of these illnesses.

By the end the year, a few cases of PCP had been reported in heterosexuals who were intravenous drugs users. Once those outside the gay community began to develop symptoms of GRID, the CDC began to suspect the disease was capable of spreading to other population groups in addition to MSM. Likewise, the fact that IV drug users were developing symptoms of GRID suggested the disease might be carried in the blood and was transferred by sharing needles.

By the end of 1981, 121 Americans had died from the disease.

1982

It was in 1982 when it was first suspected that a sexually-transmitted agent might be one of the ways GRID was spread to others. Also in 1982, the CDC first reported that HIV/AIDS was showing up in hemophiliacs and Haitians living in the U.S. Once the disease began manifesting in other population groups in addition to MSM, the name GRID became obsolete.

As a result, the name of this disease was changed to AIDS: acquired immune deficiency syndrome.

Toward the end of the year, a few previously healthy children who were given blood transfusions were found to have compromised immune systems and were starting to develop symptoms of AIDS.

By the end of 1982, there was an American dying of AIDS every day.

1983

This was the year it was discovered that HIV/AIDS could be passed heterosexually from male to female.

Because the cases of HIV infection in hemophiliacs continued to increase dramatically, the CDC warned blood banks it was likely the blood supply was tainted with the virus that was causing AIDS.

Starting in the 1960s, hemophiliacs began to benefit from the blood clotting properties of a product called Factor VIII. However, to produce Factor VIII, blood from hundreds of individual donors had to be pooled. This meant that a single donation of HIV infected blood could contaminate a huge batch of Factor VIII. This put thousands of hemophiliacs all over the world at risk of HIV, and many subsequently became infected with the virus.

By the end of the year, 3,000 new Americans were reported to have AIDS, and a thousand of them had died.

1984

Scientists finally discovered HIV, the virus that causes AIDS. Also in 1984, cases of full-blown AIDS started to appear in the U.S. in those who were infected through heterosexual intercourse.

1985

The FDA approved the first HIV antibody test to be used to determine if someone was infected with the virus. The blood banks in the U.S. finally began screening donated blood for the virus.

The news that Rock Hudson, one of America's most famous actors, had AIDS was on the front page of all major newspapers on Sunday morning, July 28, 1985. Hudson died on October 3, 1985. He was the first major public figure known to have died of AIDS, and his infection and death shocked and terrified the nation.

Also making the news in 1985 was Ryan White, a 13-year-old hemophiliac who contracted the disease from an HIV-infected blood transfusion. He became a national symbol of the intolerance of AIDS victims when school officials banned him from classes after learning he had HIV.

1986

In March of this year, while having lunch with my best friend, Dennis, I learned he was infected with the virus that causes AIDS. Six months later, in September, I was tested and learned I was also HIV-positive.

In October 1986, the U.S. Surgeon General, C. Everett Koop, published *"The Surgeon General's Report on Acquired Immune Deficiency Syndrome."* Koop's publication on the AIDS epidemic was the first publicly released report with specific information on HIV/AIDS and prevention.

The Reagan administration prohibited Koop from speaking publically on HIV/AIDS from 1981 until his report was released in 1986. Despite the administration's five-year silence on the issue, Koop believed it was the surgeon general's responsibility to inform the public about all major health issues. In his report, Koop recommended AIDS education for children *"start at the earliest grade possible."* Koop advocated abstinence as the best method for preventing transmission of HIV/AIDS, but he also strongly urged the widespread use of condoms in an effort to slow the spread of the disease.

By the time Surgeon General Koop's report was released, approximately one million Americans were already infected with HIV and 27,000 Americans had either died or were dying of AIDS.

Within a year of Koop's report, the Secretary of Education, William Bennett, apparently decided to focus on ideological preaching instead of public health. Bennett's 28-page pamphlet, which was approved by the Reagan administration, appeared to directly challenge a number of recommendations made by Surgeon General Koop, especially about teaching youth about the use of condoms to prevent HIV infection.

Bennett's booklet suggested that schools and parents teach teenagers to refrain from engaging in intercourse and downplayed the use of condoms. Critics of Bennett's booklet considered his approach to be moralizing and condemned his emphasis on abstinence, noting that by age 17, nearly half of all teenagers had already engaged in sexual intercourse.

1987

The FDA approved AZT, the first drug for treating HIV/AIDS. In clinical trials, AZT was shown to slow down the ability of the virus to reproduce in the cells of the immune system.

Even though the U.S. government was well aware of America's AIDS epidemic in 1981, President Ronald Reagan did not make his first public comments about the disease until May 1987. By the time Reagan delivered his speech on AIDS, more than 36,000 Americans had been diagnosed with AIDS, and over 20,000 of them had died. At the time of Reagan's speech, literally hundreds of thousands of Americans – perhaps as many as a million or more – had already been infected with HIV.

1988

This was an especially sad year for me. My best friend, Dennis, died of Pneumocystis carinii pneumonia in June and my "kid brother," Kenny, died from complications of AIDS in October.

The World Health Organization (WHO) declared the first World AIDS Day on December 1, 1988. World AIDS Day is now an annual event held every December 1.

Surgeon General C. Everett Koop mailed "Understanding AIDS" to 107 million households in the U.S. This eight-page booklet provided detailed advice on how to protect oneself from HIV/AIDS.

1989

The FDA approved pentamidine mist for use against Pneumocystis pneumonia. Also in 1989, the FDA authorized the use of Erythropoietin for the treatment of severe anemia, suffered by those taking AZT. Severe anemia, a side effect of AZT, was an early indication to those with HIV/AIDS that anti-retroviral medications, used to slow the progression of the disease, would potentially have a number of serious side effects.

1990

President Reagan publically apologized for virtually ignoring the AIDS epidemic while he was in office.

At age 18, in April of 1990, Ryan White died from PCP. Named in his honor, Congress passed "The Ryan White Comprehensive AIDS Resources Emergency (CARE) Act which is one of the federal government's largest health care programs. The Ryan White CARE Act provides funds for treatment, housing and other assistance to those living with HIV/AIDS who have no health insurance and limited income.

1991

The red ribbon became the international symbol of AIDS awareness. The Worldwide Health Organization (WHO) reported that 10 million people worldwide had HIV/AIDS and the number of Americans with the disease was more than one million.

Magic Johnson, one of the biggest stars in the NBA, publically announced he was HIV-positive.

The CDC reported in November that the number of AIDS cases in the U.S. had reached 200,000, having doubled in just the past two years.

1992

The first combination drug therapies to treat HIV/AIDS were introduced when the FDA approved the use of a new HIV drug, DDC, to be used in conjunction with AZT. Taking more than one drug to fight HIV was found to be more effective than taking a single drug. In addition, combination drug therapies appeared to slow down the ability of the virus to develop drug resistance.

1993

The number of Americans dying each year from complications of AIDS surpassed 40,000 for the first time.

1994

The number of AIDS cases in the U.S. doubled again to 400,000. AIDS became the leading cause of death in Americans ages 25 to 44.

1995

I contracted PCP in October. While I was hospitalized, I had a dream telling me I would begin my mission to save others from HIV/AIDS. When I was released from the hospital, I had a CD4 count of zero and was officially diagnosed with full-blown AIDS.

The FDA approved Saquinavir, the first of a new classification of powerful drugs called protease inhibitors. Protease inhibitors cause defects in newly formed HIV. These defects prevent the virus from having the ability to infect additional cells in the immune system.

More than 48,000 Americans died from AIDS in 1995.

1996

Starting in late 1995, some of those with HIV/AIDS began taking a combination of drugs including Saquinavir and other HIV drugs that were available at the time. Taking a protease inhibitor along with two or more additional HIV drugs is officially called "Highly Active Antiretroviral Therapy" (HAART). This combination drug therapy regimen is commonly referred to as someone taking a "cocktail" of HIV drugs.

By the end of 1996, the combination of antiretroviral medications used in HAART was shown to be highly effective in slowing down HIV's ability to destroy the body's immune system.

It was reported by the Joint Nations Programme on HIV/AIDS that the disease was more widespread than previously thought. The report projected that as many as 30 million people may be living with HIV/AIDS and that 16,000 people are newly infected with HIV every day.

I started HAART therapy in the spring of 1996 and my health started to improve. Later in the year, I told my story to my first two groups of teenagers – approximately 25 total teens enrolled in "at risk" classes at a local high school. The two classes were comprised of youth with previous drug, alcohol or sexual problems.

1997

The CDC reported that, for the first time since the AIDS epidemic began in 1980, there was a dramatic decrease in AIDS related deaths in the U.S. The number of Americans dying from the disease in 1997 dropped to 23,000, less than half the number of deaths that occurred in 1995.

The decrease in deaths occurred because combination drug therapy slowed down the progression of HIV to AIDS. In addition, combination therapy helped those who already had full-blown AIDS **(me)** experience improved health. As a result, those infected with HIV/AIDS suddenly began to live longer, healthier lives.

By the end of 1997, approximately 22 million people worldwide had HIV and 6.5 million had died from the disease. Most of those living in developed countries had access to care. However, the vast majority of the 22 million were in poorer, developing countries and very few of them had access to HIV medications.

1999

By this year, 33 million people were infected with HIV worldwide, and 14 million had died from the disease.

2000

The CDC reported that drug-resistant strains of HIV were being transmitted to some newly infected individuals.

2002

WHO reported that HIV/AIDS was the leading cause of death worldwide for those ages 15 to 59.

2003

Approximately 5 million people were newly infected with HIV in 2003, the largest number infected in a single year since the beginning of the epidemic. Three million people died from complications of AIDS that same year. The total number of people living with HIV/AIDS worldwide was estimated to be 40 million.

WHO and UNAIDS started a program called the "3 by 5 Initiative" to provide anti-retroviral drugs to three million people living in developing nations by the year 2005. President George W. Bush announced PEPFAR, a five-year $15 billion plan to fight HIV/AIDS internationally, primarily in Africa and the Caribbean.

2006

The CDC revised HIV testing recommendations and new guidelines advised routine HIV testing for all individuals 13 to 64 years of age.

2007

The CDC released estimates that 565,000 Americans had perished from complications of AIDS since the start of the epidemic in 1980.

2008

The CDC released its updated estimate of the number of Americans who contract HIV each year. **Current estimates are that approximately 56,000 additional Americans are infected with HIV every year. This revised number is 40 percent higher than the previous estimate of 40,000 new cases of HIV annually.**

The 20th anniversary of World AIDS Day took place in 2008. Revised estimates put the number of people worldwide who are living with AIDS at 33 million.

Today

According to the AIDS Clock (www.unfpa.org/aids_clock), somewhere in the world a person is infected with HIV every 12 seconds, and every 16 seconds someone dies from AIDS. When I checked the clock (Memorial Day – May 30, 2011) the number of those infected with HIV worldwide totaled 36,913,670.

The AIDS Clock website is made available online by UNAIDS. This organization also publishes the *"UNAIDS Global Summary of the AIDS Epidemic."* Here are a few of the summary's latest statistics for you to ponder:

- 45 percent of new HIV infections occur in young people ages 15 to 24

- 50 percent of new HIV infections occur among women

- 16.6 million children have been orphaned because their parents died from AIDS

CHAPTER 9

"Patient Zero"

In the early 1980s, most Americans, including those in the medical field, considered the new immune disease spreading across the nation to be a "gay disease." After all, the earliest victims in the country were gay or bisexual men. Remember, the medical community initially nicknamed the disease "gay cancer" based on the emergence of a number of cases of Kaposi's sarcoma in the gay community. Once the CDC realized that a number of gay men with depleted immune systems also were stricken with PCP, the term "gay cancer" was replaced with GRID – Gay Related Immune Deficiency. Yes, it was true, in the early years of the epidemic, most Americans considered AIDS to be a gay disease.

However, if you examined everyone infected worldwide during the early years of the epidemic, you would have never made the assumption the disease had anything to do with sexual orientation. In the 1980s, it was estimated that 85 percent of those infected were heterosexual. Only 15 percent of those infected worldwide were homosexuals.

Why the discrepancy? Why were the majority of those infected with HIV in America (and in Canada) during the early years of the epidemic primarily gay men? Why did the disease not appear to have a connection to sexual orientation in the majority of cases reported worldwide?

In the U.S., HIV established a foothold in the gay community before the virus spread into the general population. How did this happen?

Consider the following illustration. If there is an outbreak of the flu, it begins in one area of the country and spreads to others. For example, if a few people in New York come down with the flu in

October, those infected spread the virus to others they come into contact with, most of whom live and work in the same city. Within a matter of a few weeks or months, thousands of New Yorkers could have the flu.

If a tourist from San Francisco flies to New York in December and is exposed to the virus, he or she, once returning to California, could spread the flu to friends, family members, co-workers, etc. Here again, within a few weeks or months, the tourist's initial case of the flu could have spread to thousands of people living in San Francisco.

In this example, the flu virus first established a foothold in New York and then spread to San Francisco. Two different populations of people, thousands of miles apart, contracted the flu because of one initial case in New York.

In 1981, when HIV first established a foothold in this country, it did so in the gay community. Like New York in our previous example, the gay community was the first to be infected.

Before the end of 1982, the CDC realized that cases of GRID were starting to appear in the heterosexual community. Like those living in San Francisco in our previous example, the heterosexual community was infected after the gay community.

Since the beginning of the AIDS epidemic, people have wondered why HIV/AIDS first infected members of the gay community in this country and not the general population, as was the case throughout most of the world. A theory commonly accepted, and one that I personally believe to be accurate, involved the sexual exploits of one person, Gaetan Dugas, referred to as "Patient Zero."

If you Google "Patient Zero," you will find a number of results discussing the theory that Patient Zero, Dugas, was personally responsible for the disease's initial flare-up in the gay community.

Many of the people who have written about Dugas' connection to HIV/AIDS and his impact on the spread of this disease in America have derived their information from research done by Randy Shilts, the author of the book, ***And The Band Played On***. Shilts had a close connection to sources at the CDC who provided him with information obtained during interviews with Dugas during the early days of the epidemic.

Dugas was a handsome, gay Canadian who lived in Toronto and worked as a steward for AIR Canada. He frequently flew international flights, including those to France, the European country where the disease was most widespread before 1980. It is assumed that Dugas contracted HIV while in Paris sometime during the 1970s, and once infected, played a significant role in spreading the virus to gay men in cities throughout the U.S. and Canada.

In addition to flying to many cities as a steward, Dugas, when not working, routinely used airline passes to travel extensively. Some of his preferred destinations included cities with large, visible, gay populations including New York, San Francisco, Los Angeles, Washington D.C., London and Vancouver. Dugas, who was charming and attractive, easily picked up men wherever he visited.

Dugas developed Kaposi's sarcoma in June 1980. It was later determined that he was the first Canadian diagnosed with AIDS.

By tracing sexual contacts, the CDC knew by April 1982 that Dugas was linked to 40 of the first 248 cases of men who had contracted the disease in the U.S. These 40 men either personally had sex with Dugas, or had sex with someone who had. Nineteen of the 40 cases were in Los Angeles, 22 were in New York and the remaining nine cases were in eight different cities throughout the country.

After discovering the link between Dugas and 40 of the first men infected with GRID, the CDC contacted him for an interview. During this interview in 1982, Dugas was asked to estimate the number of his previous sexual partners. He disclosed that since becoming sexually active 10 years earlier, at age 19, he had been sexually involved with approximately 250 men each year. He "conservatively" calculated the number of his sexual partners in the previous ten years to be 2,500.

Even after the CDC informed Dugas in 1982 that he might be spreading the disease to others through unprotected sex, he refused to take precautions or make changes in his behavior. Dugas claimed the CDC had no proof he was infecting others, and he had the right to do whatever he wanted with his body. Many paid the price with their lives for his arrogance.

In March 1984, Dugas, age 31, died as a result of kidney failure caused by numerous AIDS-related infections.

There is little doubt that Dugas played a significant role in spreading the HIV/AIDS epidemic to gay men in New York and Los Angeles, where the disease was first noticed, and also to at least eight other cites in the U.S. and Canada. In the opinion of many, Dugas' flagrant promiscuity within the gay community is the primary reason the AIDS epidemic in Canada and the U.S. surfaced in that population first.

What if Dugas had been heterosexual? What if he had been sexually involved with 250 women each year rather than 250 men? If this had been the scenario, the initial outbreak of the disease in the U.S. and Canada would have occurred in the heterosexual community rather than the gay community. HIV/AIDS would never have been perceived as a "gay" disease. In my opinion, it was a fluke, a twist of fate, that MSM were infected with HIV before the general population.

Even though HIV established an initial foothold in the gay community of the U.S. and Canada, and then later started to infect the general population, the facts are that the risk of infection now exists for everyone without regard to sexual orientation.

Today, 30 years after the epidemic began in the U.S., each year more than 56,000 Americans are newly infected with HIV/AIDS and 18,000 Americans die of AIDS. According to the CDC's 2010 estimates, approximately 53 percent of those newly infected with HIV each year are men who have sex with men (MSM). Heterosexual transmission accounts for 31 percent of new infections. Injection drug users represent most of the remaining newly infected Americans, approximately 16 percent of the total infected.

The majority of the new cases of HIV/AIDS continue to appear in MSM. However, the percentage of those infected in the heterosexual community, along with IV drug users (most of whom are heterosexual), is nearing 50 percent. As the years continue to pass, it is likely the percentage of those infected in the heterosexual community will continue to rise.

Comments About "Patient Zero"

"Dear Mr. Carrel ... I do not personally have HIV, but I do have three friends whose life it has claimed in the past three years. Being gay, my chance of contracting HIV is on my mind and abstinence is the only way. I did not choose to be this way, I just am." – Bryan

"Dear Don ... I learned that homosexuals aren't to blame for starting AIDS. My father has always blamed HIV/AIDS on homosexuals, so thank you for clearing that up for me." – Spencer

"Dear Don ... Before you came to talk to us, I was unaware of how many heterosexual people have AIDS. Unfortunately, I was just one of the many that thought HIV and AIDS was mostly a disease among gay men." – Sarah

Dear Don ... I was not aware that AIDS could be transmitted through heterosexual as well as homosexual relations. I also never completely understood the origin of AIDS in the U.S. The background information that you gave us about patient zero was very informative. Thank you once again for taking your time to help educate our freshman class at SME about the consequences of unprotected sex." – Michael

"Dear Don ... I am glad you pointed out the fact that this is not a homosexual disease. It is a common misunderstanding that should be corrected." – GJ

"Dear Don Carrel ... I didn't know that 85 percent of the people in the world who are infected are heterosexuals. I thought that many more gay people were infected. Being gay myself, and just coming out, it gave me a new outlook on life. I also learned that (as dumb as it sounds) condoms are up to ninety-eight percent effective, if used correctly. My close friend Steven and I have met a boy not even 22 with HIV. My sexually active friends get tested every six months and always wear a condom. I am so proud of them." – Brian

"Dear Don Carrel ... At Sunday school we were talking about AIDS and my teacher said that mostly homosexuals get it. I thought that people would be smarter than that. I told them about you and that the majority of people in the world with AIDS are not homosexual." – Meredith

"Dear Don ... I learned that this disease is not, and never has been, the fault of gays." – Erin

"Dear Don ... I'm glad that you told everyone about how AIDS is not a "gay" disease. People can be really ignorant sometimes and it's good for them to know that. They are so quick to judge, too. It gets irritating. To me at least." – Sidney

"Dear Don ... What I didn't understand before your presenta-

tion was why homosexual people were blamed for AIDS break-ing out. I thought it was horrible and didn't make any sense. Obviously, it is still ridiculous, but now I know what the expla-nation behind that was. I'm sorry that you've had to go through so much pain in your life, but you're still here for a reason, and I'm so glad for that." – Emily

CHAPTER 10

HIV/AIDS Statistics

Finding current HIV/AIDS statistics can be frustrating. The newest UNAIDS Global Summary of the AIDS Epidemic, while recently released, is comprised of data from 2007. In addition to being outdated, statistics may vary greatly depending on the source, since statistics are often estimates, which may or may not be accurate.

For more than a decade, the CDC pegged the annual number of new infections of HIV in the U.S. at 40,000. However, after higher than expected numbers of new cases of AIDS were diagnosed, it became apparent the 40,000 estimate was too low. As a result, the CDC recently increased the estimate of new yearly cases of HIV to 56,000.

These new, higher estimates tell us that not only does HIV/AIDS continue to be a serious problem in the U.S., it is actually a larger one than the CDC suspected.

During the last decade, worldwide, new HIV infection rates are estimated to have dropped by 20 percent. Based on the CDC's recently revised estimates, the new HIV infection rates in the U.S. have not dropped 20 percent in the last decade; in fact, it would appear they have increased by 40 percent.

Worldwide Statistics

<u>UNAIDS latest Global Summary</u>
<u>of the AIDS Epidemic:</u>

• The number of people living with HIV/AIDS has risen from 8 million in 1990 to 33 million today

• Approximately 50 percent (15.5 million) of those infected are women

• 2.7 million people were newly infected in 2007

• Approximately 7,500 people are infected every day

• 2 million people died from complications of AIDS in 2007

• 25 million people have died since the pandemic began in 1980

• In Sub-Saharan Africa, where the pandemic first began, 22.4 million people are currently living with HIV and the epidemic has orphaned more than 16 million children

• 75 to 85 percent of all cases of HIV worldwide have resulted from heterosexual intercourse

Worldwide less than 40 percent of people with HIV are aware of their status. Based on this estimate, there are 20 million people who are HIV-positive and have absolutely no idea they are infected with the virus. In 1996, when I first began telling my story to others, 90 percent of those with HIV, worldwide, had not been tested for the disease and were not aware they were infected. Thankfully, worldwide, HIV/AIDS awareness is on the rise and many more people are making the decision to be tested.

U.S. Statistics

According to the Centers for Disease Control (CDC):

- In 2010 the number of new HIV infections in the U.S. was estimated to be 56,300

    - 25 percent of new HIV cases occur between the ages of 13 and 19

    - 25 percent of new HIV cases occur between the ages of 20 and 25

    - Women account for 27 percent of new HIV infections and 25 percent of those living with HIV/AIDS

    - Injection drug users represent 12 percent of new HIV infections and 19 percent of those living with HIV/AIDS

    - Men who have sex with men (MSM) represent 53 percent of new HIV infections and 48 percent of those living with HIV/AIDS

    - Individuals infected through heterosexual contact represent 31 percent of new HIV infections and 28 percent of those living with HIVAIDS

- Currently, more than 18,000 Americans die of AIDS each year

- Since the beginning of the AIDS epidemic, approximately 600,000 Americans have died from complications of AIDS

- It is estimated that 1.2 million Americans are currently living with HIV/AIDS

Note: I have seen this figure estimated to be as high as 1.9 million from other sources.

Statistics - People of Color

Unfortunately, in the U.S., HIV/AIDS statistics for people of color are even more alarming than those of the average American. According to the CDC:

• African Americans who make up only 12 percent of the U.S. population, account for almost half (47 percent) of Americans with AIDS, and 45 percent of those newly infected with HIV

• In Washington, D.C., where 54 percent of the population is black, one in 20 adults is now HIV-positive

• During their lifetime, one in 16 African American men and one in 30 African American women will be diagnosed with HIV

• The rate of new HIV infections for black men is six times higher than white men, nearly three times that of Hispanic/Latino men, and more than twice that of black women

• The HIV infection rate for black women is nearly 15 times higher as that of white women and nearly four times higher than Hispanic/Latino women

• The rate of new HIV infections among Latino men is more than double that of white men and the rate among Latino women is nearly four times that of white women

• Of the 1.2 million Americans currently living with HIV/AIDS:

    • 34 percent are white
    • 47 percent are black
    • 17 percent are Hispanic
    • 1 percent are Asian
    • 1 percent are Native Americans

Racial origin does not automatically make anyone more or less likely to contract HIV. Poverty is the primary cause of the increased HIV prevalence among African Americans and Latinos. One-fourth of African Americans live below the poverty line, a condition associated with an increased vulnerability to HIV infection. People with inadequate incomes are more likely to experience discrimination, illiteracy (resulting in less opportunity to learn about HIV prevention), drug addiction (which increases the risk of HIV infection) and sexual exploitation (rape, prostitution, etc.). Poverty is also a major factor in determining the type and quality of care available. African Americans and Latinos are more likely to be medically underserved than white Americans.

When I made the decision to write this book, I intended for the content to apply to everyone – people of all ages, races, cultures and religions. HIV/AIDS does not discriminate and can infect anyone.

However, if you happen to be a person of color, I recommend you take a close look at the statistics listed above. They clearly indicate that new HIV infections, as well as new cases of AIDS, are increasing in the communities of people of color. In North America, AIDS was originally perceived to be primarily a gay disease. If the current trend continues, in the not too distant future HIV/AIDS will be perceived as primarily as a disease of people of color. As someone who understands the hassle and high cost of HIV/AIDS treatment, it concerns me a great deal that due to economic circumstances, people of color are far less likely to have health insurance to help cover the cost of treatment.

If this trend is going to change, it is vitally important for the leaders in minority communities, including the churches, to take an active lead in promoting HIV/AIDS education and prevention.

Statistics - Youth

Young people in the U.S. are at persistent risk for HIV infections and the risk is especially notable for youth of minority races. In 2004, 4,883 Americans between the age of 13 and 24 were diagnosed with full-blown AIDS with 55 percent of those being African American youth.

Young women, especially those of minority races are increasingly at risk for HIV infections through heterosexual contact.

In America, 25 percent of all new cases of HIV occur in those age 19 and younger; 50 percent of all new cases occur in those age 25 and younger.

With 50 percent of all new HIV cases occurring in teenagers and young adults, the need for comprehensive sexual education, including specific information about how to avoid the risk of infection from all STDs is sorely needed.

Statistics - The Gay Community

In the early years of the AIDS epidemic in America, HIV/AIDS predominantly affected gay men. Men having sex with men (MSM) are still at high risk of HIV infection. According to the CDC, one in five sexually active gay and bisexual men currently has HIV/AIDS. Sadly, 44 percent of MSM who are infected with HIV have not been tested and are unaware of their positive status.

Particularly at risk are younger MSM and MSM from racial minorities. Younger MSM did not witness the tragic demise of their friends in the early years of the epidemic and, as a result, are increasingly complacent about practicing safer sex. They also remain at much higher risk of encountering a sexual partner who is HIV-positive than members of any other group in America. This is because 53 percent of those currently living with HIV/AIDS in the U.S. are MSM.

However, over the years, epidemiological patterns have gradually shifted. According to the CDC, in 2010, heterosexual transmission accounted for 31 percent of all new HIV cases – up from 3 percent in 1985.

If you take the percent of the heterosexual community contracting HIV sexually and add the heterosexuals who are infected through IV drug use, approximately 42 percent of the new HIV infections in the U.S. each year are occurring in the heterosexual community. This percent has increased dramatically over the last 20 years and it appears it will continue to do so.

Could you be an HIV statistic and not know it?

According to the CDC, approximately one-quarter of Americans infected with HIV are not aware they have the virus. HIV infection can be "silent" for a decade in most people. A substantial number of those with HIV are tested only after they develop one or more symptom of AIDS, which occur in the late stage of the illness.

If 1.2 million Americans currently have HIV/AIDS – which I believe may be a conservative estimate – then 300,000 people are walking around the streets of the U.S. infected with HIV with no idea they are capable of transmitting the virus to others.

Personally, I wonder about the accuracy of the CDC's estimate that only 25 percent of Americans with HIV are unaware they are infected. **I know very few heterosexual Americans who have ever been tested for HIV. I know very few MSM who have not been tested.**

HIV/AIDS has devastated the gay community in the last 30 years. Most MSM are well aware they are at risk for the disease, and many are tested on a regular basis. Yet, the CDC estimates that 45 percent of MSM who are positive have not been tested and are unaware of their status.

Unlike the gay/bisexual community, the disease has had less impact on the heterosexual community. It has been my experience that few heterosexuals see the need to be tested for HIV. Many hold the belief that it "can't happen to me."

The number of Americans with HIV/AIDS is expected to continue to increase over time, as antiretroviral treatment prolongs the lives of those who are infected and more people become infected with HIV than die from the disease each year. As the number of people living with HIV grows (prevalence), so does possibility for HIV transmission to others. AIDS prevalence will continue to increase, as long as the number of people with a new AIDS diagnosis exceeds the number of people dying each year.

In spite of the large numbers of deaths which have already occurred in America, and in spite of the even larger numbers of Americans who are now living with HIV or AIDS, the media-led complacency continues. Many people in the U.S. continue to think that

AIDS is something that could never happen to them. Thus, many people in the U.S. continue to become infected.

Comments: Statistics

"Dear Don ... The thing that I got out of your presentation is the fact that AIDS will drain you of your relations, money and your happiness. The impact of your presentation was huge. I am well aware of the growing percentage of people being infected with AIDS, and the statistics scare me." – Anthony

"Dear Don ... The facts scare me a lot, knowing that in about 20 years, you won't be able to have sex without there being a very high risk of getting exposed to HIV. I know that there already is a risk of contracting HIV every time you have sex, but it will increase dramatically as time goes on. When the day comes when I make the decision to have sex, I will avoid the disaster and use a condom." – Adam

"Don ... What hit me the hardest was how many people have this virus and don't even know they are infected and are innocently killing people they love." – Kristi

"Dear Don ... Growing up I had heard the disease mentioned from time to time but never had an understanding of just how destructive it truly is. I found it scary how the rate of infection is climbing fastest in teens, women and people of color." – Allison

"Dear Don ... Thanks for coming to our high school. One thing I learned is that one out of 99 people in the world between the ages of 15 and 59 is now infected with HIV. To me that is really bad because it means people are having sex at a very young age." – Lucas

"Dear Don ... You made it very clear that anyone could get AIDS. In our last school newspaper my friend told me that she read that over 80 percent of our school is sexually active. I believe it's true." – Aubrey

"Don ... One thing that I learned that I know I will always remember, and think about all the time, and will always have it in the back of my mind is how many people with AIDS don't even know that they have it. I didn't know that. It was very shocking and really scary." – Mary

"Mr. Carrel ... One thing I learned about HIV/AIDS that I didn't know before was that it is becoming more and more frequent in African Americans. This impacted me most because I am African American, so I feel like I have to be extra careful. You helped me understand how serious and dangerous AIDS really is." – Kevin

"Dear Don ... It really scares me to think that the numbers of HIV/AIDS cases in teens is growing so rapidly. What you are doing is very important and by speaking to teens, I hope that we will see these numbers drop sometime in the near future. ... One of the best ways to prevent the spread of AIDS is education, and I am afraid many of us have not had enough." – Nicole

"Dear Don ... From your speech, I learned many statistics about HIV/AIDS, and I really don't want to become one." – Evan

"Dear Don ... It's so scary to think about all those people who have no idea they are HIV-positive. I know somebody whose older brother got HIV from a drug needle. He didn't know he had it until he got the warning signs for AIDS. He's okay, but it's so sad because he's only 21." – Jessi

CHAPTER 11
HIV Testing

If you ever have had sex, especially without a condom, or you've shared a needle during drug use, you should be tested for HIV. **Both you and your partner should be tested for HIV, and learn the results, before engaging in any sexual behavior.**

The Centers for Disease Control (CDC) recommends that **everyone should know whether or not they're infected with HIV because there can be advantages to this knowledge.** If you're HIV negative, you can take steps to make sure you stay that way. If you find you are infected with HIV, you can get treatment to significantly improve your health and extend your life. If you have HIV, you also can take precautions to protect your partners. Most people who discover they're HIV-positive do change their behavior in order to reduce the chance of passing the virus on to others.

The CDC recommends a teenager as young as age 13 consider having an HIV test if he or she has been sexually active. Federal guidelines allow anyone 13 or older to be tested for HIV without parental consent. According to the CDC, 47 percent of high-school students reported having sexual intercourse at least once, and 37 percent of sexually-active students did not use a condom during the last act of sexual intercourse. More than half of all HIV-infected adolescents have not been tested and are unaware of their infection.

Personally, I believe the CDC's estimate that more than half of all HIV-infected teenagers are not aware of their infection is a conservative one. In my opinion, the rate may be closer to 90 percent. Why? My experience has shown me that teenagers rarely decide to be tested for HIV, and in most cases only do so when discovering one of their previous partners is infected with HIV.

In 1996, shortly after I started my HIV/AIDS prevention work with adolescents, I spoke to about 20 students enrolled in a health class at Blue Valley Northwest High School in Overland Park, Kansas. About a week after my presentation, I received a letter from one of the students in the class. In his letter, the student said, *"Don, thanks for talking to my class about AIDS, you should talk to the whole school ... no one in my high school thinks it's even possible they could get HIV."* He went on to tell me about one of his best friends who had graduated from BVNW the previous year and rather than attend college like most of his peers, decided to join the Marines. During the induction physical, his friend was tested for HIV. (The military routinely includes an HIV test in all induction physicals.)

To his friend's surprise, the test results were positive. His friend did what anyone who discovers they're infected with HIV should do. He went home and called all the people he had had been sexually involved with in the past and said, *"I'm sorry to have to tell you, but I just found out I'm HIV positive. You might want to go get tested."* When all was said and done, five other teenagers learned they also had HIV. Even though all five teenagers had engaged in a risky behavior resulting in their infection, none of the five realized they might possibly have contracted HIV until their phone rang.

When I received this letter from one of the first teenagers who ever heard my story, I was shocked. The students at BVNW are primarily from upper-middle class, well-educated families. It was 1996, and, at the time, it was unthinkable that a teenager from an affluent suburb would have HIV. This letter helped me understand why "the messenger" saw the need for me to tell my story to others in an attempt to save lives. This letter was the first of many from students telling me about friends and family members who actually had HIV/AIDS.

In the U.S., 25 percent of those newly infected with HIV are youth ages 13 through 19. Encouraging HIV screening in adolescents is one of the best ways to raise HIV awareness.

Surprisingly, people age 50 and over now make up 15 percent of new HIV cases. The retirement community is experiencing one of the fastest increases in the rate of new HIV infections that occur in the United States each year. Doctors rarely address sex with their older patients, and older patients sometimes have limited knowledge about HIV. Many older people aren't aware they're at risk for HIV or other STDs. Women who have gone through menopause aren't concerned with the risk of pregnancy and are less likely to insist their partners wear a condom. In addition, men are remaining sexually active at older ages due to Viagra, Cialis and other drugs, which help prolong sexual vitality. **It's imperative that everyone who is sexually active, regardless of age, be aware of his or her HIV status.**

It's also crucial that all pregnant women are tested for HIV as early in their pregnancy as possible. Prior to the mid-1990s, it was common for an HIV-positive mother to transmit the disease to her unborn child. However, it is now well documented that pregnant women with HIV who take HIV medication during their pregnancy, deliver their child by C-section and don't breast-feed their babies (HIV can pass from mother to child in breast milk) have a greater than 98 percent chance of having healthy, non-infected babies.

All major metropolitan areas have clinics offering free or low-cost HIV testing. If you're in a rural area, more than likely your county health department will have HIV testing available or be able to suggest a site where you can be tested. You also can locate the HIV testing site nearest to you by calling CDC-INFO 24 hours a day at 1-800-CDC-INFO (800-232-4636) or 1-888-232-6348 (TTY).

Some HIV testing clinics offer **anonymous testing.** When you're tested anonymously, you're not required to provide your name, address or phone number. A number is assigned when you arrive at the clinic and you must present your number to pick up your test results.

All HIV testing clinics have **confidential testing,** where the results are confidential, but you must provide your name when being tested. It is common for clinics to draw a small amount of blood to test on your first visit, and then ask you to return in person at a later date to pick up your results. Results are usually available within seven to 14 days after testing.

Rapid HIV tests are now available at many testing sites. Rapid testing normally requires only a drop of blood, often taken by a finger stick. Results are normally available within 20 to 30 minutes.

If you and/or your partner decide to be tested for HIV, it's important that you're aware it takes some time after an exposure to the virus for your test to accurately reflect your HIV status. **If you're infected with HIV one day, an HIV test will not show you're infected the next day.**

Most HIV tests measure the antibodies your body makes against HIV. It takes time for the immune system to produce enough antibodies for the test to detect, and the time required can vary from person to person. The majority of people will test positive within two to eight weeks (the average is 25 days) after the infection occurs. If you're tested three months after becoming infected with HIV, there is a 97 percent chance you will test positive. However, in rare cases, it may take up to six months to develop enough antibodies for HIV to be detected.

As I mentioned earlier, there are two primary reasons you should be tested for HIV if you believe there's even a slight risk you've been exposed to the virus either sexually or through IV drug use. First, if you're HIV-positive, you will want to know so you can take all the precautions necessary to ensure you don't infect someone else. Second, if you're infected, you should begin medical treatment as soon as possible, before the virus has substantially compromised your immune system. Starting medical treatment early may help ensure you live a longer, healthier life.

In 1986, when my doctor broke the news to me that I was HIV-positive, he walked into the room and with all sincerity, said, *"Don ... I suggest you get your affairs in order. Based on what we know about this disease today, you will be sick within a year and will more than likely die within two."* In 1986, there were no medications available to treat anyone with HIV, and at that point, it was common for those diagnosed with the virus to die within two or three years. In the 1980s, HIV/AIDS was considered a fatal disease, a "death sentence" for those infected.

Today there are a number of medications that have been developed which make it more difficult for the virus to multiply. As a result, it takes longer for HIV to destroy the immune system. However, it's important to begin treatment **before** HIV has seriously damaged the immune system. With proper care, most individuals with HIV who are diagnosed early can expect to live 20 to 30 years or more. HIV/AIDS is now considered a chronic illness similar to diabetes. Learning you're HIV-positive is no longer considered to be a death sentence.

If you are aware that you have HIV and start early treatment, in addition to living a longer, healthier life, there's growing scientific evidence showing that HIV-positive individuals who take antiviral HIV medications are far less likely to transmit the virus to others.

It is common for doctors to recommend patients with HIV/AIDS have a variety of lab tests done every 90 days. Two of the lab tests commonly recommended include one to check the CD4 count and another to check the "viral load." These tests help to determine the extent of immune system damage HIV has caused and to indicate the speed at which the virus is multiplying. For example, a person with a normal, healthy immune system might have a CD4 count of 1,100. The virus progresses by destroying T-cells, which in turn causes the CD4 count to decrease. The closer the CD4 count gets to 200, the more likely the individual will develop an opportunistic (potentially deadly) infection. Someone who is living with HIV is reclassified as someone living with AIDS, once his or her CD4 count is below 200 and an opportunistic infection has occurred.

A viral load test indicates how rapidly the virus is making progress in its war against the immune system. When the viral load test result is classified as "undetectable," HIV is typically not making progress in destroying one's immune system. If the viral load is undetectable and the CD4 count is increasing rather than decreasing, it would indicate the immune system, if anything, was improving.

A growing number of studies have been done indicating that if an individual's viral load is undetectable and the CD4 count is stable, the chance the infected individual will transmit HIV to someone else is significantly reduced. **However, someone with an undetectable viral load should never assume it's not possible to infect his or her partner.**

If you're sexually active and single, I recommend you and your partner be tested for HIV on a regular basis, preferably every six to 12 months. Always keep in mind that a "negative" HIV test result means the person was definitely HIV free six months ago and more than likely not infected three months ago. However, a result from a test taken today may not yet show infection that occurred from an exposure to the virus within the last three months.

The following are behaviors that increase your chances of getting HIV. If you answer yes to any of them, you should definitely be tested for HIV. According to the CDC, if you continue with any of these behaviors, you should be tested yearly.

- Have you injected drugs or steroids or shared equipment (such as needles or syringes) with others?

- Have you had unprotected vaginal, anal, or oral sex with men who have sex with men, multiple partners or anonymous partners?

- Have you exchanged sex for drugs or money?

- Have you been diagnosed with or treated for hepatitis, tuberculosis (TB) or a sexually transmitted disease (STD), like syphilis?

- Have you had unprotected sex with someone who could answer yes to any of the above questions?

If you have had sex with someone whose history of sex partners and/or drug use is unknown to you or if you or your partner has had many sex partners, then you have more of a chance of being infected with HIV. Always remember that **both you and your new partner should be tested for HIV before having sex for the first time.**

Everyone should know whether or not they have HIV. If you and your partner have been tested and are both HIV negative and you both remain faithful to each other (monogamous) and don't have other risks for HIV infection, then you will not need another HIV test unless your situation changes.

Comments about HIV Testing

"Dear Don … I'm not sure if your goal was to scare us straight or not, but you sure did that to me! I want to thank you for that most of all. I'm 16 and have been sexually active for over a year now, my current girlfriend is the same. Neither of us have been tested, and neither of us were virgins when we met. I'm going to go get tested and make her go, too. I know she won't want

to, and I know she'll say no at first, but now I feel that it is very important to do, even though I'm terrified of what the test might reveal. Thank you for showing me the light." – Josh

"Dear Mr. Carrel … I learned so many useful facts and now know that the only way to truly stay away from HIV/AIDS is just not to have sex. I know that you might have changed some people's lives because I know many who went to get an HIV test." – Alex

"Dear Don … I knew someone with HIV. He ended his life on his own. The last time I saw him he looked great and was really happy. I found out he was HIV positive in February after he killed himself. I met him a year earlier. To make a long story short, I was drunk and ended up having sex with him. I had two HIV tests that both came back negative. Since then I have never taken another drink. If my test had come back positive I hope I could do what you are doing. You have such an impact on people." – Sally

"Dear Don … You have opened my eyes and now I see how dangerous sex and drugs can be. I have always known them to be that way but now there is a whole different meaning to dangerous. Many of my friends talked to you last Friday and decided to go get tested. That, to me, is very awesome." – Tabitha

"Dear Mr. Carrel … What you said affected me so much that I'll never look at having sex the same way again. My friend and I are going to go and get checked (tested) next week. I am glad you can share your inspirational story with so many people. I hope you can save many young people like me from making stupid mistakes. … You were put on this earth for a reason and I believe heaven's gate will be wide open for you. You have affected my life greatly and I will never forget your visit." – Brian

"Dear Don … Two teenagers get HIV every hour. That's really scary. I've been involved in 'risky' behavior. Each time I had sex it was unprotected. The only thing I was really worried about was getting pregnant. I didn't even think about getting HIV. I thought of STDs, but didn't worry about them. I know at least two out of the four guys I've slept with have had multiple partners. Now, I'm scared I might be sick. I want to get tested, but I don't want to tell my mom. Plus, I'm really scared the results might turn out positive." – Lindsay

"Dear Don … I haven't exactly made the safest choice because I just lost my virginity a couple of weeks ago and I am going to go get checked for AIDS because I would rather know so if I do, I won't pass it on. I'm praying I won't. I am so scared my Dad will find out because he always thinks of me as his little angel. I am; I just made a bad choice." – Kara

"Don ... You've changed my mind a great deal. I am sexually active with my boyfriend right now. I have only had sex with my current boyfriend and one other guy in the past. My past boyfriend had many partners before me and assured me he was disease free. Your presentation encouraged me to get a test and check for myself. I want to thank you for overcoming any shame or embarrassment you have about having AIDS and coming to tell your story. You changed one 17-year old girl's life." – Megan

CHAPTER 12

Treatment of HIV

In the earliest years of the AIDS epidemic, there was no treatment for HIV; the disease had nearly a 100 percent mortality rate. Those of us diagnosed in the 1980s were told we could expect to live only a few years. In 1987, the first drug to fight HIV, AZT, was approved by the FDA. Since then, many medications have been developed to treat the disease.

New treatments have slowed the progression from HIV to AIDS, and from AIDS to death for people infected with HIV. Consequently, both AIDS cases and deaths have dropped dramatically, and an increasing number of people with HIV are living longer, healthier lives. HIV/AIDS is no longer considered a fatal disease. As mentioned earlier, it is now a chronic disease, similar to diabetes.

According to a study published July 26, 2010, in *The Lancet*, the average life expectancy for a 20-year-old, living in an industrialized country who never contracts HIV is an additional 60 years, with death occurring, on average at age 80. Someone of the same age, who is HIV-positive and begins antiretroviral medications (ARVs) while still 20, can expect to live 11 years less, on average to age 69.

The February 1, 2011, issue of *The Journal of Infectious Diseases* reported that 30 percent of all people who enter HIV care for the first time have CD4 counts below 200, and a significant percentage of them have a CD4 count under 100. HIV-positive people who don't start ARVs until their CD4 levels drop to 100 are expected to live 10 years less (to age 59) than those who started therapy when their CD4 counts were above 200.

The above studies illustrate the importance of beginning treatment for HIV/AIDS as soon as possible after infection occurs. If you believe there is **any** chance you've been exposed to HIV, you should be tested as soon as enough time has passed to ensure the test results are accurate. If you learn you're HIV-positive, it's important to begin treatment before the virus has had time to do serious damage to your immune system.

If you learn you are HIV-positive, schedule an appointment with a physician who is not only an infectious disease (ID) specialist, but is also well versed in the treatment of HIV/AIDS. Determining the proper drug regimen to effectively treat the disease is complex and ever changing. Failure to obtain treatment from someone who keeps abreast of the rapidly changing treatment options could result in a much shorter life expectancy.

In addition, I recommend you look for an ID specialist who favors starting ARV treatment immediately. U.S. guidelines, as of the summer of 2011, recommend treatment should begin when the CD4 count drops below 500, but some doctors don't follow standard guidelines and start treatment later. There are many doctors who agree with my opinion that treatment should begin sooner than current guidelines.

According to an article published by AIDSMEDS (www .aidsmeds.com) on May 12, 2011, the results of a major international study, funded by the National Institutes of Health (NIH) may persuade doctors to offer medication as early as possible. The nine-nation study conducted on nearly 1,800 HIV serodiscordant couples, in which one partner is HIV-positive and the other is HIV-negative, found that by starting ARV treatment early, HIV-positive partners were **96 percent less likely to spread the virus** to their uninfected partners. All but one of the couples studied were heterosexual couples. In this study condoms remained crucial for protection, and all of the couples in the study were urged to use them.

Half of the study's HIV-infected partners started medication immediately after diagnosis and the other half delayed taking ARVs until his or her CD4 levels dropped below 250 or symptoms of the disease began to appear.

Over the length of the study, there were 28 couples where the uninfected person became infected. Only one of the 28 couples was from the group where the HIV-infected partner started treatment early. The group of couples where treatment was delayed contained 27 of the 28 cases where HIV was spread to the uninfected partner.

This cannot be overstated: If you believe you could have been exposed to HIV/AIDS, you should be tested. **Current research indicates that those who are HIV-positive will live a longer, healthier life if treatment is not significantly delayed. In addition, those with HIV who begin ARV treatment as soon as possible have a much lower chance of transmitting the virus to others.**

Once infected with HIV, it may take as long as eight to 12 years, sometimes longer, for the virus to damage someone's immune system to the point that he or she develops physical symptoms of the disease. If treatment is delayed until symptoms appear, the immune system will already be seriously damaged. Those starting ARV medications at this point will be far less likely to have a life expectancy near that of someone who never contracts HIV.

The development of many different ARVs to prolong life for those with HIV/AIDS is a great achievement. I would've died many years ago without new medications that were introduced in the 1990s. However, the improvements in treatment have unfortunately resulted in some unforeseen adverse consequences.

Starting in the mid-1990s, when many HIV-positive Americans began ARV therapy, the death rate for AIDS decreased dramatically. The press faithfully reported the latest details about new treatments and enthusiastically reported statistics showing lower death rates. As a result of this extensive coverage, many people began to believe HIV/AIDS was no longer a serious problem.

Most of the people I speak with today are aware the death rate for AIDS has dropped dramatically. It has not only been widely reported in the press, but the disease is far less noticeable than it was 15 years ago. Before the introduction of ARVs, it was common to see people with AIDS (PWAs) in public. They were often extremely thin, "looked sick" and appeared to be dying. Because of improvement in care, PWAs in such sad, physical shape are rarely seen today. As a result, the disease is now mostly invisible to the public.

Unfortunately, those who are aware the AIDS death rate has decreased often assume it must also mean less people are contracting HIV. This assumption is not only false, but the opposite is true. More, not fewer, Americans are contracting HIV than ever before.

A lower death rate for AIDS does not correlate into a lower infection rate for HIV. In 1995, before combination therapy was introduced, approximately 48,000 Americans died from complications of AIDS, and it was estimated that 48,000 additional Americans were newly infected with HIV the same year. By 1997, new medications were extending the lives of those with HIV/AIDS, and only 23,000 Americans died from the disease that year. This number was less than half of the deaths that occurred in 1995, two years earlier. However, in 1997 the number of those newly infected with HIV remained similar to the number of those infected in 1995. **The death rate decreased dramatically, but the infection rate did not.**

In 2010, the death rate was even lower, 18,000 Americans died from AIDS. However, those newly infected with HIV in 2010 are estimated to be between 56,000 and 60,000.

Most Americans don't realize that HIV/AIDS prevalence (the number of Americans who are actually living with HIV) is increasing every year. In 2011, it's estimated that **at least** 1.2 million people are walking around the streets of the U.S. with HIV/AIDS. In 1997, there were approximately half as many Americans living with HIV/AIDS as there are today.

Besides the increase in HIV/AIDS prevalence, the improvement in care has resulted in another **frightening repercussion.** There's a growing perception among many sexually active youth that contracting HIV is not a "big deal" anymore. After all, if you're infected, all you have to do is "take a pill or two and everything will be all right." This attitude is especially true in the younger gay community where there has been a significant increase in new infection rates in recent years.

I place a great deal of the blame for this lack of concern on the press, which frequently reports the success of new HIV treatments but rarely, if ever, puts any emphasis into reporting the cost of these medications or the many, often serious, side effects associated with taking them.

Newer, simplified treatment

At one point a few years ago, I swallowed 38 pills every day and had an injection every 12 hours. I was once on a drug regimen that required I take some medications twice a day, some three times a day; some had to be taken on an empty stomach and others had to be taken right after eating. Trying to figure out what to take when was a nightmare.

Over the last 20 years, treatment for HIV/AIDS has become much simpler. Current drug regimens require HIV medication be taken only once or twice daily, and in many cases two or three different ARVs have been combined into one tablet so those with HIV are taking much smaller "handfuls" of pills than in the past.

Cost of HIV medications

One of the first things someone diagnosed with HIV/AIDS learns when starting treatment is that having HIV is expensive. In addition to the cost of medication, it's common for a "healthy" HIV patient to have doctor and laboratory bills of well over $10,000 a year. The cost of treating HIV/AIDS often drains the financial resources of those with the disease, and many die in poverty. A surprisingly large number of PWAs are not only poor, but also homeless.

"Dear Don ... I didn't realize that people who suffer from AIDS would likely end up dying in poverty. I didn't realize the amount of money that's necessary for medication, doctor's visits and other expenses. I know that for myself, I'm not going to have sexual intercourse with anyone but my wife and your talk has fortified my belief for not participating in sexual activities until I'm married." – Brad

I recently printed a list from my health insurance company showing the cost of my prescription medications for 2010. **In 2010, the total cost of my medication was $49,765 for the year. This breaks down to an average of $4,147 a month; $138 a day.** My medication costs in 2010 were relatively low compared to a few years ago when the cost was $250 per day or $91,000 for the year. Thankfully, the majority of the costs for my prescription drugs are covered by my insurance. Unfortunately, one out of every six Americans has no health insurance to pay for medications.

If you are newly diagnosed with HIV, don't panic. Your initial drug costs won't be nearly as high as mine.

Currently, newly infected individuals beginning medical care for HIV are commonly prescribed three different ARVs. Many long-term survivors, like me, take more than three ARVs because our virus has become increasingly immune to treatment. I currently take five ARVs to slow the progression of my virus. In addition, I must also take a number of medications necessary to counteract long-term side effects of HIV/AIDS treatment.

Recently, I questioned my HIV doctor, an infectious disease specialist at KU Medical Center in Kansas City, about what combination of drugs she typically would recommend for someone starting treatment shortly after being infected with HIV. According to my physician, one of the most common drug regimens currently used for a new patient would consist of a single pill called Atripila. This

HIV medication is a combination of three ARVs (Sustiva, Emtriva and Tenofovir) formulated into one pill. The recommended dosage of Atripila is one tablet, taken once daily. Obviously, this drug regimen is extremely easy to follow. After all, what could be easier than taking only one pill, once a day?

I checked with my pharmacy on the cost for a month's supply of Atripila and learned that the current charge would be $2,056 for a one-month supply, or $24,672 for the year. This amount is half the current cost of my prescription bill, but even so, most people would be shocked to learn how expensive it is to purchase this bottle of medication containing only 30 tablets.

Hopefully, if you are newly infected with HIV you have health insurance to help cover the cost of treatment. However, even if you have health insurance, it rarely covers the entire charge. Most policies have co-pays requiring the insured to pay part of the cost. In addition, many health insurance policies have yearly or lifetime limits on the amount of coverage. For example, a policy may cover up to $10,000 in prescription drugs a year and require the insured to pay any charges over the $10,000 limit. If you're taking Atripila and your insurance company has a $10,000 annual limit for prescription drugs, your insurance would pay $10,000 of your annual cost of $24,672. You'd be responsible for the $14,672 difference.

Almost all industrialized countries in the world have universal health insurance to cover the health care costs of every citizen. Unfortunately, Americans don't have universal health coverage. The U.S. government has been debating the pros and cons of universal health coverage for many years, but no such program currently exists. Based on the current political climate, it seems unlikely universal coverage will be available in the U.S. for many years. **As a result, approximately 47 million people, nearly one out of every six Americans, have no health insurance.**

In addition to having 47 million uninsured Americans, the majority of those with health insurance are insured by group plans connected to their employment. Coverage could be lost, or drastically reduced, if the person becomes unemployed or decides to retire.

"Dear Don ... Another thing I learned was about all the medications needed to be taken to stay well, and how expensive they are, especially to those who have no insurance, are jobless or bankrupt. That to me sounds unfair and makes me so

outraged, because it's like the government is practically shout-
ing "Oh, hey! Look! This person has almost no money left and
will die sooner than they need to and suffer more if they don't
get their prescribed meds that cost more than they can afford,
but oh well, I don't care.' This is completely wrong! People with
HIV and AIDS did not ask for it, they just got it." – Lee Ann

Several government programs exist to assist those with
HIV/AIDS by paying the high costs of the medications they need to
stay alive. The AIDS Drug Assistance Program (ADAP) and the
Ryan White CARE Act are two of the best known of these programs. They both help HIV-positive people without private insurance cover the cost of prescribed AIDS medications. However, both
have stringent eligibility criteria based on the amount of income the
person earns. The annual income of those receiving assistance
must be extremely low. Anyone making what most would consider
a "middle-class salary" would not qualify for assistance. In addition,
there are often waiting lists to receive assistance because of limited
available funds. Those with HIV may have to wait for months or
years before receiving the drugs they need to remain healthy and
alive.

People with HIV/AIDS struggle daily with emotional and sometimes physical symptoms of the disease. Improvements in HIV
treatment definitely have resulted in those with HIV living longer.
However, the longer someone with HIV lives, the longer they must
struggle with the emotional stress associated with having the disease. Those stresses include concern about paying the high and
ever-increasing cost of their HIV treatment. Even those like me, who
are fortunate enough to have health insurance, continually worry
about what would happen if they were to lose their insurance coverage.

In 1995, when I was treated for PCP, the total cost for my treatment exceeded $100,000. Fortunately, I had health insurance, pur-
chased 12 years earlier, and most of my medical expenses were
covered. Several years later, I received a letter notifying me the
company I had been insured with for years was "going out of business and cancelling all their health coverage nationwide." I was
given six months to find new insurance – an impossible task for
someone with full-blown AIDS.

Unbelievably, within a few months of losing my insurance coverage, my partner's company made the decision to offer health

insurance to the domestic partners of its employees. The company initially offered "open enrollment" where you could apply for the insurance without answering any medical questions – without regard to pre-existing conditions. The timing and availability of this health coverage was a miracle and one I'm extremely thankful for. If I had permanently lost health insurance coverage, I have no idea how I would cover the cost of my medical treatment today.

I have often wondered if "the messenger" played a role in making sure I had continued access to health care.

Even though I was lucky enough to obtain insurance through the domestic partnership program offered by my partner's employer, I still worry that I could lose this coverage at any time. If my partner stops working for his company tomorrow, either because he is terminated or decides to leave voluntarily, my health insurance would end immediately. If my partner had a job offer with a higher salary or greater future opportunities, he might be unable to accept the offer unless the company making the offer also had domestic partnership coverage available. Unfortunately, very few companies in the U.S. do.

Many people with HIV/AIDS who are employed and have health insurance are often "trapped" in jobs they don't enjoy. They are unable to change jobs if it results in the loss of their health insurance. HIV-positive workers who earn an income low enough to qualify for medication provided through ADAP or the Ryan White CARE Act often must refuse promotions that would raise their income above the limit eligible for assistance. A raise in pay isn't likely to compensate for losing access to a program paying for thousands of dollars worth of HIV medication.

It's true: if you're HIV-positive and have the means to obtain medication you can expect a longer, healthier life. However, the ability to pay for treatment is a life-long concern for anyone with HIV/AIDS.

Comments: HIV Medication

"Dear Don ... I was shocked when you showed us the amount of medicine required and how much it cost. The disease truly takes over every aspect of your life." – Mark

"Dear Don ... What impacted me the most about your presentation was the size and the amount of pills that you have to take daily. It is remarkable to me how incredibly expensive your medication is, and it makes me sad to think about how many infected people there are that cannot afford treatment." – Sarah

"Dear Don Carrel ... I was very interested in learning about how many medications you have to take and how expensive it is. I had no idea that you had to change medications every year or so because of mutation." – Allie

"Don ... After watching your presentation one thing stuck out in my mind and that was how much your medicine cost. I am trying to get a car at the moment and if I had to pay for the meds, I would never be able to get it. ... No one should ever have to make the choice between letting their family eat or buying a drug that could save their life." – Patrick

"Dear Don Carrel ... I think that it is very cool that you are using your life to help protect us kids. I always knew that HIV could be deadly, but I never imagined it being so expensive. I mean I couldn't even believe all the pills that you have to take every day. When I take my vitamin in the morning I think that is a lot. I would never be able to swallow some of those pills. Well, I think that it is pretty cool that you have been so strong through all the years. I hope you stay well, and congrats on the grandchildren." – Matt

"Dear Don ... I actually learned a lot of things from you coming and speaking. I thought I knew kind of a lot, but I knew absolutely nothing, according to what you said. I was shocked when told us your medication costs $80,000 a year. I was also shocked to learn how many people are infected and have absolutely no clue that they have HIV." – Morgan

"Dear Don ... I had no idea the medications could take that great of toll on one's bank account, but it is obviously very hefty. I was curious though; does insurance not cover at least some of the expense? And why is it so expensive? I feel that after your talk, I'll take a second thought before ever having unprotected sex again." – Henry

Side effects of medications

The press gives even less attention to the side effects of HIV medications than to the excessive cost of treatment. Taking ARVs has been described as undergoing "retro-viral chemotherapy." If someone is treated for cancer, he or she normally feels lousy due to the unpleasant side effects of chemotherapy. Anyone HIV-positive who's taking ARVs normally feels lousy. The biggest difference is that undergoing chemotherapy for cancer doesn't last forever. If you have HIV, you take ARVs forever.

Most people on HIV medications have at least some mild to moderate side effects. In general, the higher the number of drugs being taken, the more side effects someone experiences.

According to AIDS Info Net (www.aidsinfonet.org), the most common side effects of HIV/AIDS medications are:

- **Fatigue** – People on HIV medications frequently are tired for at least part of the day.

- **Anemia** – Anemia causes fatigue and is a marker that increases your risk of getting sick with HIV infections or other illnesses.

- **Digestive Problems** – Many HIV drugs can make you sick to your stomach. They can cause nausea, vomiting, gas or diarrhea. Diarrhea can range from being slightly inconvenient to a severe, debilitating condition.

- **Lipodystrophy (Body Shape Changes and Facial Wasting)** – A number of HIV medications cause fat loss in arms, legs and face, or fat gain in the stomach or behind the neck.

- **High Levels of Fats and Sugar in the Blood** – ARVs can cause increases in cholesterol, triglyceride and glucose, which increase the risk of heart disease, heart attack, stroke and diabetes.

- **Skin Problems** – Some ARVs cause rashes. Most are mild and often temporary, but in some cases they can be serious. Other problems include dry skin and hair loss.

- **Neuropathy** – Neuropathy is a painful condition caused by nerve damage, which normally starts in the feet or the hands.

• **Mitochondrial Toxicity** – This condition damages the structure inside the cells. It can cause neuropathy or kidney damage and a serious buildup of lactic acid in the body.

• **Osteoporosis** – Osteoporosis frequently shows up in people taking ARVs. Bones can lose their mineral content and become brittle. A loss of blood supply can cause hip problems. I'm personally acquainted with a number of HIV-positive individuals who've had one or both hips replaced because of severe pain and difficulty walking due to deterioration of their hip joints.

• **Sexual Dysfunction** – A significant percentage of HIV-positive people, possibly as high 75 percent, experience some form of sexual dysfunction, including decreased libido (sex drive), trouble getting or maintaining an erection and the inability to ejaculate or experience an orgasm. Erectile difficulties are common, especially in the first months following diagnosis. These may be related to worries about transmitting the disease to a partner. Difficulties with premature or delayed ejaculation, largely due to psychological issues, can also appear. Various physical factors can also contribute to erectile dysfunction. These include problems affecting the cells that line the inside of penile arteries, diabetes, neurological disorders such as multiple sclerosis or hormone imbalances such as low testosterone.

If you look at the list of the potential side effects of Atripila, the drug that currently is often recommended for someone newly infected with HIV, you'll discover that taking a single tablet of this medication each day can result in one or more of the following complications:

• Memory loss, trouble concentrating and hallucinations
• Severe depression, paranoia, anger and thoughts of suicide
• Fatigue
• Rash – mild to serious
• Liver problems, including liver failure or death
• Thinning of the bones, bone pain and fractures
• Muscle weakness and muscle pain caused by kidney problems
• Upset stomach, nausea, vomiting and gas
• Feeling cold (especially in the arms and legs)

- Dizziness, headache, trouble sleeping, drowsiness
- Fast or irregular heartbeat
- Jaundice, yellowing of the skin
- Loss of appetite
- Changes in body fat

It's difficult to believe the side effects listed above can result from taking only one Atripila tablet each day – at a cost of $2,056 a month. If you're one of those people who believes that contracting HIV today is not such a "big deal" because you can "take a pill or two and everything will be all right," you might want to reconsider your opinion.

The "joys" of my treatment

Early in my mission to help prevent others from contracting HIV, I learned that facts and figures are rarely remembered and have little impact on changing attitudes or behavior. People remember real stories about real people. The story about my HIV treatment is one I remember all too well.

"Beep, Beep, Beep – Beep, Beep, Beep"

In 1988, two years after I learned I was HIV-positive, I began taking AZT, my first antiretroviral medication. At the time, the recommended dosage of AZT was between 1200 and 1500 mg daily, an amount considered dangerously high by today's standards. AZT often causes terrible side effects, the worst of which is severe anemia.

When I started AZT, I was prescribed 1200 mg daily and the monthly cost was $1,100. Not long after I started the drug, I began to notice that it dramatically affected my energy level. I was constantly exhausted, which made it extremely difficult to put in the hours required to manage *Kitchens Plus* and *The Croissant Café*, my two businesses.

When the FDA first approved AZT, it was widely believed that keeping the level of the drug in your bloodstream constant was vitally important to ensure it was effective. Those taking AZT were instructed to take two capsules every four hours. According to those manufacturing the drug, the doses needed to be "exactly" four hours apart or the drug's level in the bloodstream would vary, making it considerably less effective in slowing the growth of the virus. The recommended schedule was two capsules at 6 a.m., two capsules at 10 a.m., two capsules at 2 p.m., two capsules at 6 p.m., two capsules at 10 p.m. and two capsules at 2 a.m. Initially, I set my alarm clock to wake me up at 2 a.m. and 6 a.m. so there was no chance I could miss taking a dosage. At the time, I remember thinking, *"If I have to take AZT, every four hours, forever, I'll never get a good night's sleep again."*

During the day, I was **constantly** checking my watch to make sure I swallowed my AZT **exactly** on time. It was a horrible reminder. Before I started AZT, I could occasionally "forget" I had

HIV and actually felt "normal" for a while. But once I started AZT, I was forced to remember, every four hours of the day, seven days a week that I was infected with a deadly virus.

A few months after I started AZT, small pillboxes with built-in digital timers hit the market. Apparently someone looked at all the people required to take AZT every four hours on the dot, invented the pillbox with a timer and made a fortune. Everyone taking AZT rushed out to buy one. I could put my AZT in the box, set the timer for four hours, put the pillbox in my pocket and wait to hear, *"Beep, Beep, Beep – Beep, Beep, Beep – Beep, Beep, Beep."*

My little digital pillbox was a lifesaver. I still had to be reminded every four hours I had HIV, but at least I no longer had to watch the clock constantly. However, there was one problem with my new pillbox. It was sometimes challenging to explain to anyone within hearing distance what was beeping.

A few months after the introduction of the "beeping" pillbox, I was in Dallas at market shopping for merchandise for *Kitchens Plus*. While I was there, I decided to take time to see Lily Tomlin, who was in town performing in a one-woman show. I was seated in the audience enjoying Tomlin's show with hundreds of others when precisely at 10 p.m., *"Beep, Beep, Beep – Beep, Beep, Beep,"* echoed throughout theater. The sound was loud enough that Tomlin stopped her performance, and somberly said something to the effect of, *"Isn't this disease a bitch?"* Obviously, there were a lot of "us" in the audience hiding pillboxes in our pockets. After that experience, I never felt quite as alone in my struggle against this disease.

From the time I started AZT in 1988, until I was hospitalized with PCP in October of 1995, I remained healthy, even though HIV was slowly destroying my immune system. Despite the fact I was taking AZT, in the fall of 1995, HIV won the battle. My immune system was annihilated.

Unless you have been skipping chapters, you already read about my battle with PCP in October of 1995. When I was released from the hospital, my CD4 count was zero. My immune system was not functioning. I no longer just had HIV; I had, and continue to have full-blown AIDS.

Within a few months of my release from the hospital, I started ARV treatment by taking a combination of three HIV drugs. Over the next six months or so, my CD4 count slowly increased and stabilized in the low 200s. It remained close to that level for the next 12 years. Once someone's CD4 count bottoms out at zero, it's extremely difficult to boost the levels beyond a certain point. Going from my deathbed with a CD4 count of zero to someone still living with a CD4 count of 200 was more than I had expected.

During the 12 years starting the end of 1995 and continuing until the fall of 2007, my health was fair, but not great. During those 12 years, I normally forced myself out of bed between 7 a.m. and 8 a.m., and I felt fairly good for the first part of the day. However, by early to mid-afternoon, I was exhausted and wanted only to sleep. Every afternoon when AIDS-related fatigue set in, I felt like some type of electrical appliance that had just been unplugged from the socket. Not only was I physically wiped out, I couldn't think clearly, and as a result, was even afraid to drive.

I spent every afternoon napping for two or three hours. After my nap, I would eat dinner, watch television, usually while in bed, and fall asleep sometime between 9 p.m. and 10 p.m. My social life was almost nonexistent. On the rare occasions I did go out for dinner or to a party, I always headed for home about 9 p.m., not because I wanted to leave, but because I couldn't stay awake.

My bout with PCP is the only time I have been hospitalized for an AIDS-related illness in the entire 30 years I've had HIV. However, I've been admitted to the hospital three times since then because of serious side effects caused by one of my HIV medications.

My first serious medication-related complication took place early in 1997. During my second date with Chris, I experienced a life-threatening, allergic reaction to a new ARV medication I had been taking for less than a month. It started with a day of diarrhea, vomiting and fever. My entire body broke out in a rash, and I turned the color of a bright, red apple. My temperature spiked to a 105. My doctor ordered me to stop taking my new medication immediately. Before leaving the hospital four days later, I was warned that if I ever took that particular medication again, the allergic reaction would be much worse and would likely kill me.

My "Roto-Rooter" surgery

My second medication-related hospitalization was one I'll not forget. I was stricken with kidney stones when Crixivan, another HIV medication I was taking, failed to dissolve completely, and I ended up with particles of drug "crystals" in my kidneys. These drug crystals caused the same type of blockage that occurs when someone has kidney stones.

Kidney stones can get stuck in the ureters (tubes that carry urine from the kidneys to the bladder) and block the flow of urine out of the kidneys. If the ureters are blocked, the kidney starts to swell, which in turn causes pain. The pain is usually severe. If you've never had a kidney stone, the pain is indescribable. On more than one occasion, I've heard women who have had kidney stones describe the pain as being far worse than childbirth.

Kidney stones normally pass on their own within a day or two, and treatment typically involves taking oral medication to control the pain until the stone passes. Occasionally, the pain is so severe as to require hospitalization where stronger pain medications can be administered until the stone passes. In a small number of cases, surgery is required to remove the stones.

Lucky me! The pain from my drug-induced kidney stones was so excruciating, I ended up in the hospital on morphine. Even the morphine seemed to do little to stop the pain. For seven days, while I waited for my stones to pass, I was in agony, constantly begging the nurses to increase the amount of my morphine, hoping to get relief from the pain. Finally, it was determined I needed to have surgery. Apparently, the crystals from Crixivan were tougher than normal kidney stones and passing them was nearly impossible.

When I first learned I was going to have surgery, I was elated. After seven days, I would have done anything to get rid of the pain. However, once the surgeon came in to explain the procedure to me, my excitement turned to trepidation. The surgery consisted of guiding a miniature light, camera and stent up the urethra and through the bladder to reach the ureter. Once there, the stent, which would widen the opening of the ureter, would be put in place and left for two or three days to give the stones time to pass.

The surgeon wanted to know if I preferred to have a local anesthetic, which would eliminate the pain, but allow me to be awake during the procedure, or if I would like to be put completely under. It was an easy decision. If he was taking a light, camera and equipment up my penis, I preferred not to be there for the experience. I chose to sleep through the procedure.

I woke after surgery and everything appeared to be okay. There were no visible signs of bruising and "everything" appeared to be normal. I felt a sense of relief, that was, until I had to urinate. It burned – so severely I literally cried out in pain, and it was the first time I had ever seen what appeared to be red urine. For the next 24 hours I'm not sure what was worse, the pain from my kidney stones or building up the nerve to empty my bladder.

To top things off, the procedure had to be repeated three days later to remove the stent. I actually can joke about it now. On occasion, I have included this story when talking about my life with HIV. I fondly describe my kidney stone episode as the time I had "Roto-Rooter" surgery.

Trying to find humor in a situation that involves pain, embarrassment or both has helped me emotionally survive AIDS. Finding humor in the worst of circumstances helps me avoid depression, which can be far worse than any physical pain.

"The sticky side always goes down"

In November 2003, my primary-care physician recommended I have a routine colonoscopy, something everyone over 50 should do. My routine colonoscopy ended up having anything but routine results. I was diagnosed with anal cancer. Later in the book, I will talk about various STDs, including HPV. HPV is the most common sexually transmitted virus in the country. It causes genital warts for males and females and may lead to both anal and cervical cancer. Unlike almost all other STDs, there is a vaccine to prevent HPV. I highly encourage both females and males to be vaccinated for HPV before becoming sexually active.

Many more people are aware of the risks of cervical cancer than anal cancer. Perhaps it's because those with anal cancer find it an embarrassing topic to discuss. Like cervical cancer, if left untreated, anal cancer can result in death. In 2009, one of America's most loved actresses, Farrah Fawcett, died from complications of anal cancer. She bravely battled the disease for three years. Anal cancer awareness increased dramatically because of Fawcett's diagnosis, treatment and subsequent death from the disease.

After my cancer diagnosis, I was referred to both an oncologist and a radiologist at KU Medical Center in Kansas City. The prognosis was anything but comforting. I had no choice but to treat the cancer, and the treatment needed to include both radiation and chemotherapy. However, because of my already seriously compromised immune system, my oncologist gave me only a 50 percent chance of surviving treatment. The odds were definitely worrisome, but I had no choice. I could not ignore my cancer or I would die.

As I was making arrangements to undergo treatment, my partner, Chris, did some Internet searching and discovered a physician, Dr. J. Michael Berry, at the University of California in San Francisco (UCSF) Medical Center who had developed a surgical procedure to treat people with anal cancer. Dr. Berry had successfully treated hundreds of patients for this disease in the last few years without the use of radiation or chemotherapy.

Chris and I made the decision to fly halfway across the country to meet with Dr. Berry. Having a surgical procedure to treat my cancer, even though it required going to San Francisco, seemed like a much safer option to me. At the time I agreed to be treated by Dr. Berry, I paid little attention to what might be involved in recovering from the procedure. If I had understood it more clearly, I may have never had the nerve to show up for the surgery.

In April 2004, Chris and I arrived bright and early one morning at the UCSF Medical Center for my scheduled procedure with Dr. Berry. The surgery required anesthesia to "knock me out," but an overnight stay at the hospital was unnecessary. In fact, Dr. Berry insisted I be on a plane back to Kansas City before the anesthesia wore off. Apparently, after it did so, I would be in considerable pain. When explaining why it was best for me to fly home immediately after the procedure, Dr. Berry smiled, and said, *"I don't want to be within swinging range once your anesthesia wears off."*

My "Roto-Rooter" surgery a couple of years earlier was a picnic compared to what Dr. Berry planned to do to tackle my anal cancer. It definitely took me a couple of years before I could make light of what I now describe as my "blow-torch" surgery.

My "blow-torch" surgery consisted of the destruction of my cancer cells by basically burning, to the third degree, the entire lining of my rectum. By doing so, the "skin" which lines the rectum was completely destroyed, hopefully along with my cancer, leaving in its place what I can only describe as completely raw tissue. Dr. Berry explained before performing the procedure that afterwards there would be *"some bleeding for the next few months"* and for the first week or so, I would experience *"mild to moderate"* discomfort when having a bowel movement.

When Dr. Berry told me to expect bleeding after the procedure, all I can say is the two of us have an entirely different opinion about the definition of what *"some bleeding"* entails. After the procedure was finished, while still too groggy from the anesthesia to comprehend or remember much, Dr. Berry suggested to Chris that we purchase "mini pads" to put inside my underwear to absorb any bleeding before getting on the plane to head back to Kansas City.

Before we left the office, a follow-up appointment with Dr. Berry was scheduled for August, four months following my surgery.

The airfare for my frequent trips to USCF was expensive enough to handle and thankfully, Chris and I never had to pay for lodging. I have three cousins – Pam, Katy and Bill – who all live in the Bay Area.

My cousin, Pam, picked us up after surgery so we could have lunch together before heading to the airport for our flight home. I was still "hung over" from the anesthesia and have no memory of lunch. However, I vaguely remember our trip to the store after lunch to pick up mini pads before the trip home. Being a male, my knowledge of mini pads was somewhat limited, and the thought of wearing them wasn't something I was looking forward to doing. My "experience" while shopping for mini pads is perhaps best described by my cousin.

My cousin, Pam

My cousin, Don, came to San Francisco on several occasions to see a specialist for treatment for anal cancer. It was an opportunity for me to spend time with my "favorite" cousin Don, and his partner, Chris.

On Don's initial visit to the doctor, he had an aggressive surgical procedure that left him bleeding for many days. Per his doctor's orders, we stopped at Safeway and the three of us trooped down the feminine hygiene aisle in search of mini pads. I was trying to go quietly as to not attract any unwanted attention to the fact I was shopping for feminine hygiene products with two men.

Don's pain meds had not worn off yet; so in his usual booming voice (he doesn't have an inside voice) he wanted to discuss the pros and cons of wings versus no wings, extra length versus regular size, super absorbent versus light days. He wanted the entire rundown.

Much to my chagrin, many passing shoppers overheard our conversation and we received a few looks of disapproval. Don looked at several of the annoyed shoppers and in exasperation, blurted out 'I just had surgery and I <u>have</u> to wear these things.' One woman was so intrigued that she joined our discussion in order to add her opinion.

After much thought Don made his selection. My last piece of advice to him was to always remember, 'the sticky side goes down.'

As funny as that scene in the grocery store was, we all knew Don was not in good shape. It made me so sad to see such a vibrant, bigger-than-life character like Don in so much pain.

When Chris and I returned to UCSF Medical Center in August 2004, four months after my surgery, I was still bleeding, still wearing mini pads and not completely healed from my surgery. Before Dr. Berry operated, he had explained that the surgery, even if successful, would not mean I was permanently cured of anal cancer. It would be necessary for me to return to UCSF for a follow-up cancer screening every three or four months, perhaps forever, if the cancer was recurring.

Even though health insurance covered most of Dr. Berry's medical charges, it did not pay for the airplane tickets Chris and I needed to make frequent trips to San Francisco. Dr. Berry insisted I not make the trip alone because some visits might involve "touch-up" laser treatments to any area that was cancerous or suspected to be pre-cancerous. Since the touch-up laser treatments in layman's terms – involved charring only part of the rectum, and not all of it, they wouldn't be as invasive as my original surgery, but could still require I have a traveling caretaker.

Since I wasn't completely healed for my August checkup, Dr. Berry was not able to tell much from my exam. We scheduled another checkup for January 2005. During my January examination, Dr. Berry discovered what appeared to be two pre-cancerous areas. He biopsied the areas and called a few weeks later to let me know the areas were indeed cancerous. While on the phone, we scheduled a date for a laser touch-up session in March 2005.

Nine days before my scheduled visit to UCSF in March, I ended up in the emergency room at KU Medical Center. I had been suffering from a sinus infection for about three or four weeks when my temperature suddenly spiked to 104. Something besides a sinus infection was definitely affecting my health. I had not felt this sick since coming down with PCP 10 years earlier.

The hospital was filled to capacity because of an enormous outbreak of the flu, and I waited in the ER for more than 12 hours before a room was available. It was after midnight when I was finally assigned a hospital room. My physician ordered a battery of tests in an attempt to find out what had caused my sudden and severely elevated temperature. It appeared I had a serious, rapidly growing infection. I was so ill my doctor wanted the tests done immediately, even though it was the middle of the night.

What seemed to be gallons of blood had already been drawn from my arm, and I was just starting to drift off to sleep when a young doctor and a younger resident came into the room and informed me they were there to give me a spinal tap. It was my first, and I hope last, spinal tap. The thought of having a needle, that appeared to be a foot long, forced into my spine in the middle of the night, terrified me. To make matters worse, as I sat on the bed shaking and leaning over to grab my ankles, I heard the doctor say to the resident, *"Put the needle right there and push hard, you'll feel some resistance when it hits the spine, but keep pushing."* I nervously glanced up at the doctor who I knew personally, and in a quivering voice inquired, *"Mark, has she ever done this before?"* His response was, *"Oh yes, many times."* I guess sometimes it does make sense for your doctor to tell a white lie.

The spinal tap was needed to rule out the possibility of a bacterial infection in my spinal fluid, which could quickly become fatal. Over the next 12 hours, I had X-rays, a colonoscopy to check for serious digestive infections, and more blood tests.

After all the tests, the results were inconclusive. I did not have a recurrence of PCP, no bacterial infection in my spinal fluid, no life-threatening case of the flu, no intestinal infections, and my blood and urine tests provided no clue as to what was wrong. It appeared I didn't have any HIV-related illness. Not knowing what was wrong or how to treat it, my doctor hooked me up to massive doses of intravenous antibiotics and hoped for the best. With my outcome uncertain, my sons, Chris and Matt, made an emergency 500-mile trip from Indianapolis to Kansas City, not knowing if it would be the last time they ever saw their dad.

After being hooked up to an IV pumping me full of antibiotics for four days, I recovered. I was released from the hospital four days before my scheduled trip to UCSF Medical Center. My physician was not supportive of the idea of my getting on an airplane and flying halfway across the country when I had just been released from the hospital after nearly dying from some unknown infection. However, there was no way I was going to reschedule my appointment. The airline tickets were purchased and I was going.

Wearing a mask over my nose and mouth to hopefully filter out germs circulating throughout the plane's ventilation system, I left for San Francisco as planned. Dr. Berry removed the two cancerous areas in my rectum with a laser. We scheduled another appointment for September, and Chris and I were back on the plane immediately after the procedure. As expected, there was more bleeding and pain, but it was nothing compared to my original "blow-torch" surgery.

Call me a "pin cushion"

In the summer of 2005, my HIV labs showed that my CD4 counts were beginning to fall, and my viral load was increasing. (A viral load test checks for the activity level of the virus. The higher the results, the faster the virus is replicating.) It was not good news. My labs indicated my current drug regimen was starting to fail. My virus had apparently mutated to the point my medications were becoming less effective. Over the years, I had already developed resistance to most available HIV drugs. I had one option left, the first drug available in a new classification of medications called fusion inhibitors: a drug called Fuzeon.

When I started Fuzeon it was considered to be "the drug of last resort." It was rarely prescribed to anyone unless all the other ARVs were no longer effective in slowing the growth of HIV. Few people with HIV, me included, would ever want Fuzeon as part of their drug regimen.

Fuzeon is an expensive medication, about $4,000 a month and it must be injected into your system every 12 hours. In addition, the side effects can be unpleasant. Ninety-eight percent of patients experience reactions at the injection site such as pain, itching, bruising, nodules, infections and redness. In addition to the above mentioned side effects, those taking Fuzeon may experience: constipation, cough, depression, diarrhea, eye infection, flu-like illness, fatigue, itchy rash, loss of appetite, muscle pain and weakness, pain and tingling in the hands and feet, nausea, nervousness, sinus problems, skin warts, stomach pain, swollen glands, trouble sleeping and weight loss. It makes one wonder if dying from complications of AIDS might not be a better choice than injecting Fuzeon into your body every 12 hours.

Too stupid or stubborn to give up – I'm not sure which – I started on Fuzeon. Even though I've been poked with a needle hundreds of times, and have had enough blood drawn over the years to fill a battleship, I'm terrified of needles. I've never watched anyone give me an injection or draw my blood. If someone on television or in a movie is about to get an injection, I shut my eyes.

Not only is Fuzeon given by injection, the drug must be injected s-l-o-w-l-y or it clumps up in knots and does not absorb properly into your system. Sticking myself was difficult enough without having to dilly-dally around and s-l-o-w-l-y push in the plunger. The only way I could bear to inject myself was to lay on the bed, take a couple of minutes to build up my nerve, jab myself in the stomach or upper thigh and hope that I didn't pass out while s-l-o-w-l-y pushing in the plunger.

Only two things saved me. First, when Chris happened to be home, he'd do the "jabbing and injecting" for me. Second, the manufacturer of Fuzeon started a research study to test the effectiveness of administering the drug with a needleless "gun" rather than a syringe. I jumped at the chance to join the study and "shoot" myself rather than continue life as a pincushion. The needleless gun, called a Biojector, forces the Fuzeon through the pores of the skin by using high pressure supplied by a CO_2 cartridge. When you pull the trigger, it releases a very fine, high-pressure stream of medication that penetrates the tiny openings of the skin, spreading out the medication as it is forced into the tissue beneath. I loved my Biojector. All I had to do was jab it in my stomach, thigh or arm and pull the trigger. When it went off, I frequently cried out, "OUCH." It felt like a bee sting, but at least it was over in less than a second. I was so grateful. My obliging Biojector did not s-l-o-w-l-y inject Fuzeon into my system; it was faster than a speeding bullet.

"Dear Don ... One thing in particular that I learned and found interesting was your medication. I was appalled to see that you had to go through all of the pills and injections EVERY DAY for the rest of your life. The cost wasn't something to grin at either." – Patrick

In September 2005, I was back at UCSF for another checkup and managed to escape the visit unscathed by both the biopsy knife and the laser. However, during my November visit, three months later, there were more biopsies, which proved to be pre-cancerous and my second laser touch-up surgery was scheduled for February 2006.

That January 2006, I made an appointment to see my infectious disease specialist at KU Medical Center. My mouth was full of what I can best describe as white "slime." I kept spitting it out, only to have my mouth quickly fill up with more slime. I had thrush. In scientific terms, thrush is a yeast infection of the mucus membrane lining the mouth and tongue and is caused by a fungus called

Candida. A small amount of this fungus lives in almost everyone's mouth, but it's usually kept in check by your immune system. However, when your immune system is weaker, the fungus can grow, leading to sores. Thrush appears as whitish, velvety lesions in the mouth and on the tongue.

In addition to treating me for thrush, my ID specialist removed three cancerous growths from my lips.

The next month, it was off to San Francisco for another laser touch-up by Dr. Berry. My summer of 2006 check-up revealed no signs of cancerous or pre-cancerous tissue. During my follow-up exam in September 2007, Dr. Berry again found no evidence of cancer, declared my rectal tissue as extremely healthy – much healthier than he had expected – and said it wasn't necessary for me to return for another check-up for a year. Things were looking up. It appeared my mini pad days could be over.

As I mentioned earlier, HIV often mutates and becomes resistant to various medications. If someone develops resistance to a specific drug or classification of drugs, it's often necessary to change his or her drug regimen. The change can be made by switching to all different ARVs, stopping one or more of the current medications and replacing them with a different one or by adding other medications to the drugs currently taken. While it's common for those taking HIV medications to take three different ARVs, long-term survivors often need to take more than three.

In 2005, when I began Fuzeon, it was only one of five different ARVs I was taking to control my HIV. Between then and the summer of 2007, the FDA approved a number of new HIV medications. Two years after starting Fuzeon injections, I was able to modify my drug regimen to include newer ARVs and stop Fuzeon. To say I was thrilled would be an understatement. Biojector or not, I do not miss pulling that trigger every 12 hours.

You must be kidding, the possibility of death?

I still take five ARVs. The more HIV medication someone takes, the more likely there will be unpleasant side effects. Almost everyone I know taking ARVs experiences some side effects and most of those consider the side effects bothersome enough that they negatively affect the quality of their everyday life.

At one point in the early 1990s, not long after I first started my drug cocktail, I picked up the first month's supply of a brand new HIV medication at the pharmacy. When I arrived home, I sat down at my kitchen table to read the list of side effects. As I was reviewing the rather lengthy list, I was shocked! Right there, in black and white, it said, side effects of the drug include "the possibility of death." It seemed unbelievable that taking a drug prescribed to help fight HIV could kill me.

Starting that day, nearly 20 years ago, I made the decision to stop reading information about the potential side effects of the drugs in my regimen.

However, for this book, I broke my "rule" and looked up the side effects associated with the five HIV medications included in my drug regimen. Listed below are the potential side effects of my current ARVs (as of July 2011).

- **<u>Five out of five</u> potentially cause:** nausea, liver, kidney or heart problems.

- **<u>Four out of the five</u> potentially cause**: diarrhea; vomiting; headache; abdominal pain (mild to severe); high sugar and fat levels and the onset or worsening of diabetes.

- **<u>Three out of the five</u> potentially cause:** fatigue; fever and chills; ear, nose or throat problems; skin rash (mild to severe); dizziness; loss of appetite; flatulence (gas); sore throat; muscle or joint aches and pains.

- **<u>Two out of the five</u> potentially cause:** jaundice (yellow eyes or skin); depression and suicidal thoughts; fat redistribution/accumulation (changes in body fat); weakness, burning and pricking sensation in the hands and feet; constipation and intestinal cramps.

- **One out of the five** potentially causes: indigestion, anemia (mild to severe); drowsiness; inflammation of the pancreas; irregular heart rhythm; lightheadedness and fainting; change in taste; sweating; pink eye; blisters and sores in the mouth.

Do these side effects impact the quality of my everyday life? I can assure you they do. I've been taking HIV medications continuously since I swallowed my first two capsules of AZT in 1988, and I've been coping with unpleasant side effects of those medications ever since.

Thankfully, I don't suffer from all the possible medical conditions that could be associated with my present-day treatment. However, I can, without hesitation, say that I have dealt with nuisances associated with well over half of them. Some days the problems are worse than others. Some days the problems are barely noticeable. Some days the problems are so annoying, intolerable or confining that my day is wasted attempting to manage them. Perhaps the biggest problem is that I never know what to expect on any given day.

"Oh, crap!"

One of the most bothersome, infuriating and often embarrassing problems associated with many of the ARVs is diarrhea. I cannot think of a single person I know with HIV, or a single friend or acquaintance who died from complications of AIDS, who has not dealt with this medication-related curse.

There was a five-year period of my life when I **never** left home without a backpack containing an extra change of clothes. On more than one occasion, I have abandoned my full grocery cart in the aisle of the store and fled when suddenly, without **any** warning, I filled my pants. The same situation has occurred on a number of times while working out at the gym, driving down the road or walking my dog around the block.

At one point in my life, I was in a support group with others living with HIV/AIDS and the "lack of bowel control" issue was one we all faced. It was frequently discussed, sometimes in tears, and occasionally with laughter.

"Don ... It must be embarrassing for you when sometimes you 'crap' in your pants because of your meds. Sorry if that's too harsh to say." – Kate

"Don ... You had a lot of courage and confidence talking to us. I could never tell a group of teenagers that I "crapped" my pants. Thanks for being so honest. It really hits homes when speaker are honest." – Patrick

Is there a cure for HIV/AIDS?

There is no cure for HIV/AIDS. However, that being said, there has been one reported instance, involving one person who has possibly been cured of HIV. According to an article by Tim Horn, posted to **AIDSmeds** and **Poz** on December 10, 2010, doctors in Berlin, Germany, treated an American, Timothy Brown, for a relapse of acute myeloid leukemia; a potentially fatal cancer of the immune system. In February 2007, Brown was given a bone marrow transplant. A German cancer specialist, Dr. Gero Huetter, and his colleagues decided that instead of simply performing a transplant to increase Brown's chance of surviving leukemia, to perform one that might also increase his chance of surviving HIV by using stem cells from an HIV-resistant donor.

Such a treatment is difficult. The person's immune system must be shut down and restarted with the new stem cells from a donor who is a perfect tissue match for the patient and has an unusual mutation called Delta-32. Delta-32 is a rare genetic defect. If someone inherits this genetic mutation from both parents, the cells of their immune system are highly resistant to HIV.

On the day Brown received his stem cell transplant, he discontinued the use of his antiretroviral medications. Approximately 13 months after the initial transplant, Brown's leukemia reoccurred and a second transplant using the rare stem cells was performed. The second treatment has, thus far, led to a remission of the cancer.

According to a detailed report published in **The New England Journal of Medicine** written three-and-a-half years following the initial transplant, Brown's CD4 count has returned to normal, well within the range of HIV-negative individuals. In addition, Brown currently tests negative for HIV. Based on these results, it is reasonable to conclude that Brown has possibly been cured of his HIV infection.

However, the odds of finding a tissue match for someone with HIV/AIDS to another person who has inherited the Delta-32 mutation from both parents is one in perhaps millions. In other words, while Timothy Brown appears to be cured of HIV at the present time, the likelihood of others with HIV/AIDS locating a match and having the financial resources to undergo this transplant procedure is nearly zero.

The bottom-line: "There is no cure for HIV/AIDS."

Will there ever be a cure for HIV/AIDS?

Currently, the best any of us can do is hope and pray there will some day be a cure for HIV/AIDS. I believe a cure will be many years in coming, and perhaps never will be found. HIV is a virus, and viruses are historically difficult, if not impossible, to cure.

While it may be possible to develop a vaccine that's effective in the prevention of some of the strains of HIV, it will be difficult, perhaps impossible, to develop one that will protect against all the mutated viruses that now exist. The relatively few different strains of HIV that originally existed have mutated over the years due to exposure to different ARVs used and interaction with individual immune systems. As a result, there are now virtually thousands of unique strains of HIV.

Why are HIV medications so expensive?

Drug companies have done a magnificent job in developing new medications to extend not only the lifespan of those with this disease, but also improve the quality of their lives. The many HIV drugs that have been fast-tracked onto the market have saved millions of lives, including my own. But those drugs, especially the newer, more effective ones, come with a prohibitively high price tag.

My pharmacy bills, labs costs and medical bills have totaled more than $100,000 a year for a number of years. I'm what could be considered a "cash cow" for the medical and pharmaceutical industries, and I'm only one of an estimated 1.2 million Americans with HIV/AIDS.

Many with HIV/AIDS have long wondered why medication that is necessary to keep us alive is so expensive. Many other people, who do not have HIV, but suffer from other medical conditions equally life threatening, have wondered the same thing. When I first began taking AZT, my monthly pharmacy bill for this one medication was $1,100. You can now purchase AZT for $34 a month or less. Why? AZT is now available in generic form. If a pharmacy can still make a profit selling AZT for $34, it obviously costs little to produce the drug. Why did the manufacturer of AZT charge $1,100 for a medication that costs almost nothing to manufacture? Perhaps it was because anyone trying to stay alive would pay the price.

Drug companies often justify the high cost of new drugs by pointing out that developing drugs is expensive, and the cost must be recouped once the drug is approved by the FDA and becomes available to the consumer. To some extent this justification is true. However, in many cases, a great deal of the cost to develop a new drug is borne by the federal government.

And, how do pharmaceutical companies justify substantial increases in the price of a drug developed many years earlier if it's subsequently learned the drug is effective in treating a different condition than for which it was originally intended? For example, early in the AIDS pandemic, the most common cause of death was PCP. Initially, there was no effective treatment for this rare form of pneumonia, and most people who contracted it died.

However, in the late 1980s, it was learned that aerosolized pentamidine was effective in treating and preventing PCP. Pentamidine was originally developed in 1941 for use in the treatment of a sleeping sickness associated with tuberculosis. Before the early 1980s, the CDC stored the nation's entire supply of pentamidine because there were so few demands for this medication. Prior to learning pentamidine effectively treated PCP, the cost of an aerosol container of the drug was approximately $11. As soon as it was learned this drug helped those with PCP, the cost of a container shot up to over a $100. Why did the manufacturer of pentamidine suddenly increase the price tenfold? Perhaps it was because anyone trying to stay alive would pay the price.

Why are drugs that are manufactured in the U.S. considerably less expensive when purchased in Canada than in America? It's because Canada has universal health care coverage and has negotiated a lower price with American drug manufacturers. Why are there laws in the U.S. prohibiting groups from negotiating lower prices for Americans taking such expensive medication?

Why are Americans often required to pay such exorbitant prices for prescription medications? Perhaps it's because anyone trying to stay alive will pay the price.

Treatment: My final thoughts

I'm grateful for the vast improvements in treatment for HIV/AIDS over the last 20 years. I have great faith that treatment will continue to improve. Looking back at my personal struggle with AIDS, and my fight to stay alive, I'm immensely thankful. I honestly can say that each time my virus mutated to the point it was too powerful to be stopped by any of the medications available at the time, science managed to unleash a new drug or a new classification of drugs that literally saved my life. Sometimes, I believe "the messenger" is watching over me and when it appears I'm in trouble, helps AIDS researchers come up with something new, just in the nick of time, to treat this disease.

However, I understand all too well that having HIV and living longer doesn't come without a price. In the 1980s, those with AIDS did not have long to worry about the cost of their medical treatment, or how to pay for it. Death in the early days of the epidemic was not without pain, but it was usually over within a few months. Those with AIDS worried about dying, but they did not have to be concerned about the long-term problems associated with living with HIV.

If you're newly infected with HIV, and you begin treatment, you'll initially only be taking a few ARVs a day and can expect to live nearly as long as your friends without HIV (perhaps 10 years less).

However, every day you are alive, you'll worry about how to pay the costs of your ever-increasing medical care. Every day you live, you may be forced to deal with what are often, unpleasant side effects of your medication.

You may be "trapped" in a job you do not enjoy. Or stuck in a career without the potential for success because you have health insurance and changing jobs would result in loss of access to your life-saving medications.

It won't be easy to date. I can assure you there are few people without HIV who are comfortable having a sexual relationship with someone who is HIV-positive.

If you have HIV and still plan to be sexually active, hopefully you would never consider doing so without revealing your status to your partner in advance of any act that would place him or her at risk. Unfortunately, some people with HIV don't feel it's their responsibility to tell their sexual partners they have HIV. Even more frightening, there are many thousands of people with HIV who are unaware they're infected. Both are reasons I encourage everyone to always assume anyone they come into contact with may have HIV.

Will you ever get married? If you have HIV, it's difficult enough to find someone to date. Most people are simply not comfortable with the concept of having sex with anyone infected with this virus. If you're HIV-positive, finding someone to date who is also willing to "fall in love" and marry may be impossible.

If you do marry, will you have children? If you're an HIV-positive male, it's difficult to conceive a child without running the risk of infecting your spouse. It's possible, if you're an HIV-positive female, to have a healthy child. However, it requires artificial insemination to eliminate the risk of infecting your male partner. Once pregnant, you must start ARVs during your first trimester, deliver your child by C-section and never nurse your child. If you follow the above guide-lines, there is nearly a 98 percent chance your child will be born without HIV. However, if you're HIV positive is it wise to have children? With the expense of your own care will you be able to support children financially? Will you remain healthy and alive long enough to raise your children?

Legally it's your responsibility to disclose your HIV status to any potential sex partner prior to taking any action that might possible put him or her at risk.

State laws for failure to reveal your HIV status in advance vary, but are often quite severe. For example, in Missouri, according to RSMO 191.677, if you have sex with someone, even if you use a condom, and fail to disclose your HIV-positive status in advance, you can be charged with a "Class B Felony, punishable by five (5) to fifteen (15) years in prison." If your partner actually contacts HIV, it's considered to be a "Class A Felony, punishable by ten (10) to thirty (30) years or life imprisonment." Violation of this law can also result in a civil action against you, punishable by fines and other costs.

In addition, your friends, family and acquaintances, who aren't infected with HIV, will be spending their disposable income on vacations, new cars and nights out on the town. You, on the other hand, might be spending your disposable income at the pharmacy. How will that feel?

While it's now possible to live a longer, healthier life with HIV/AIDS than those stricken early in the AIDS pandemic, it is no reason to be less concerned about contracting the disease. Living a longer life with HIV is forever challenging.

Long-term HIV survivors face a number of medical, financial and emotional problems. According to the American Academy of HIV Medication, HIV survivors 55 and older are three times as likely as non-infected 70-year-olds to suffer chronic heath problems: hypertension, diabetes, osteoporosis, heart disease and cancer to name a few. Hip replacements and severe fatigue occur much earlier in life than with non-infected individuals. Long-term HIV patients are 13 times more likely to suffer from depression than the average American. Older HIV/AIDS patients are also much more likely to be unemployed, short on savings, living in poverty and homeless.

I said it before, but it definitely bears repeating. "If you're one of those people who believes that contracting HIV today is not such a 'big deal' because you can 'take a pill or two and everything will be all right,' you might want to reconsider your opinion."

CHAPTER 13

HIV Prevention

It's a fact that you can virtually eliminate your risk of contracting HIV/AIDS by abstaining from sexual activities and avoiding the use of IV drugs. While I always stress abstinence during my presentation, it's also a fact that the majority of high school students participate in some type of sexual activity before they graduate.

According to the CDC, nearly 75 percent of teenagers have had sexual intercourse before the age of 20. Because of the prevalence of sexual activity in youth, discussing the advantages of abstinence-only sex education doesn't help protect teens who already are sexually active from contracting HIV or other risks associated with premarital sex. As a result, this chapter also will discuss in detail how to minimize risk through safer sex.

Most adults, including myself, do not believe unmarried teenagers should be having sex. However, we're not the ones who decide when someone will make the choice to become sexually active. The individual always makes that decision. Anyone old enough to make the choice to have sex, whether it's wise or unwise, should have access to education explaining the risks involved, as well as the steps he or she can take to reduce those risks. It's my sincere belief that starting in middle school and continuing into high school, all students should have access to comprehensive sex education.

By comprehensive sex education, I mean the information presented should stress the advantages of abstinence and provide detailed information about the risks involved in sexual activities and how to reduce those risks by having safer sex.

Before those of you who believe in abstinence-only sex education take me to task, I have something for you to ponder. When my parents were married in the 1950s, they were teenagers. When I married in the early 1970s, I was in my early 20s. When my sons married, they were in their late 20s. The trend today is to marry later in life. Many couples don't say, "I do" until they're in their late 20s, 30s or even older. Do you honestly believe those of all ages will abstain from sexual activity until marriage? As I said earlier, anyone old enough to make the choice to have sex deserves access to comprehensive sex education.

Often, those involved in sexual education, including parents, discuss the subject in general terms and fail to give specific information about what can be done to prevent unwanted pregnancies and STD infections. In this chapter, you'll find I've included explicit details and some content that may shock you. In an effort to help others avoid HIV/AIDS, and other consequences that might result from risky behavior, I would rather provide too much detail than not enough.

"Dear Don … Now every time I hear the words HIV, AIDS or sex I will think of you and what you taught me. I'm so glad you talked about sex because I had questions but I would never ask my parents because we don't talk about sex at my house. Luckily, you came and answered them." – Jessica

Abstinence

If you would like a 100 percent guarantee that you'll never contract HIV/AIDS, it's really quite simple. Never have sex with anyone. Never share a needle with anyone or participate in any other activity that results in blood-to-blood contact. Simple advice, but realistically, few of us will practice abstinence for life.

However, if you want to avoid contracting HIV at this point in your life, don't share needles and always practice abstinence. *"Abstain from sex."* I know, if you're a teenager, you've heard this before – from your parents, teachers, clergy and maybe even your friends.

Whenever I speak, I never preach about abstinence, because it's not my decision to make. Whether or not you choose to be sexually active is your decision, not mine. However, in every presentation I always say, *"Knowing what I now know about AIDS, and how it has impacted my life and the lives of so many of my friends, if I could snap my fingers and trade places with you, a high-school student who does not have HIV, I can guarantee that you would never find me in the back seat of my car some Saturday night risking my life for 15 minutes of fun. Knowing what I know now, if I were a high school student, I would abstain."*

My comment about *"risking my life for 15 minutes of fun"* always makes those who hear it stop and think. **Regardless of your age, you should seriously consider whether or not having sex at this point in your life, with this particular person, is worth the possible consequences.**

Comments: "15 minutes of fun"

"Hi Don ... I learned a lot about HIV and AIDS. I learned that 15 minutes of fun is not worth a lifetime of sickness. I also learned that when or if you get HIV/AIDS, you don't have to lose hope." – *Greg*

"Dear Don ... I want to tell you that you're pretty brave to get up in front of thousands and thousands of teens like myself and get in our heads that this disease is not worth 15 minutes of party time with someone else." – *Cathy*

"Dear Don ... My mind was thinking differently about sexual relations after I heard your speech. I thought it was all fun and

games, but then the consequences come into play and then you are in a world of hurt." – Nick

Despite the recent surge in abstinence-only programs, experts say that most teenagers will break their pledges to abstain before they're married. On the plus side, a number of studies show that teenagers who make "virginity pledges" wait an additional 12 months before having vaginal intercourse and also tend to have fewer partners than those who have not agreed to remain abstinent until marriage.

However, many of those same studies show that teenagers taking abstinence pledges are less likely to use condoms once they do become sexually active. Additionally, those taking pledges have an increased likelihood of substituting oral or anal sex for vaginal intercourse ("real sex"). Participating in these two "not real sex" activities puts participants at a higher risk of contracting STDs. As a result, teens in abstinence-only programs have a higher rate of STD infection than those who receive comprehensive sex education.

When it comes to sexually transmitted diseases, the U.S. offers woefully inadequate education. The CDC reports that 19 million new STD infections occur every year. Even more alarming is that nearly 50 percent of these infections are in young people between the ages of 15 and 24. It's apparent that many of these STD statistics could be reduced with proper education. Abstinence-only education fails to teach measures to use during sex to protect oneself from STDs.

These statistics are frightening and help illustrate the need for comprehensive sex education that encourages abstinence and provides detailed information on how to reduce sexual risks by having safer sex. At some point in time, those who choose to abstain will reach a point in life where a sexual relationship becomes a priority. He or she should have the knowledge needed to make safer choices when that time comes.

Comments: Abstinence

"Mr. Carrel ... you possibly could have saved me from ruining my abstinence plan. I never considered what a person with this disease goes through everyday of their life." – Mary

"Dear Don ... The fact that you want to share your story and make sure others don't end up in your shoes is really cool. I am 15 years old and I am proudly, still a virgin. I am a virgin in a world full of sex and peer pressure, but I know how to say no. Most of my friends have already had sex, and after your talk I think they all are going to get tested. ... Your personality is a reflection of your bravery. You are just as real as your disease." – Alex

"Dear Mr. Carrel ... Your story brought tears to my eyes. ... There are some of my very close friends in my class that are sexually active. They do it a lot and most of the time it's protected, but there have been exceptions. I have never seen them worry about anything other than pregnancy, but yesterday I think you opened their eyes and showed them that it can happen to anybody. Now I'm not the only one worried about them. They are worried about themselves as well. As for me, I have chosen to abstain and save my virginity until marriage. Your talk yesterday made me proud of my decision. I get a lot of grief and flack for being a virgin. Sometimes I question my decision, and then I realize that I'm only 16 and not ready to be a mother, not ready to get married and certainly not ready to die. I've been thinking a lot the last 24 hours about what you shared with us. What you are doing is wonderful. Not only does it help to change sexually active people's minds, but you reassure people like me that abstinence is the safest sex." – Michelle

"Dear Don ... You have definitely given me, a person who has already decided to try my best to abstain from sex, an even stronger reason to wait. I have always been aware of the potential of becoming infected with HIV and AIDS, but never really thought about it all that much. The numbers and statistics are startling. I never realized how many people are infected and don't even know it. There should be more people out there like you, trying to make people more aware." – Adam

"Dear Don ... I am only fifteen years old and I was not thinking about having sex anytime soon. Now, after hearing your speech about real life situations, I feel that I should totally abstain until marriage. ... I definitely do not think I will have sex in high school, thanks to you." – Holly

"Dear Mr. Don ... What opened my eyes was when you explained how lonely AIDS really is, and how it destroys all your hopes and aspirations ... I've decided to wait to have sex and to think about the consequences. Not just from parents and adults, but also that just by doing one thing you think is cool could kill you." – Carly

"Dear Don ... Personally, I found your speech to be very compelling, motivational and influential. I know that I will abstain from having sex now after hearing what you had to tell us. ... It was very motivational to see a man like yourself not afraid to

discuss and explain to us how HIV/AIDS has affected his life. You delivered not only a message that taught us about the virus itself, but one of compassion and understanding that allows us to see how not only how the victims of this disease are affected, but how their family and friends are as well. You have encouraged me to stay away from risky behaviors and I will do everything I can to remain HIV/AIDS free." – Jacob

"Dear Don ... My uncle died of AIDS-related cancer a few years ago. After taking this class and listening to you, I feel abstinence is the best way of life for me at this time. I also would like to state that I respect you very much. Through all the misery in your life, you still see meaning." – Bret

"Hi Don ... Rather than reprimanding us and tell us what we should and shouldn't do, you simply made us aware of the consequences of certain actions we might take. I, myself, feel that abstinence is the best form of safe sex. I'm planning not to have sex until I am married; your talk only reinforced my feelings." – Becky

"Dear Don ... You changed my whole outlook on life. I am a born again virgin. My girl friend is a natural virgin. So I'm going to try to stay with her as long as I can. Your presentation was tight. I felt you provided a lot of information for the class and broadened our awareness of AIDS." – Greg

"Dear Don ... I'm 14 and I'm not sexually active and I don't plan to now that I heard your speech. It was very good for you to talk about what happened to your friend. Now I'm very scared about HIV and don't plan to get it." – Laura

"Dear Don ... I'm only 14 years old (In my mind I'm going on 21). I've been practicing abstinence since I can remember. Though this year I almost let my guard down because I saw my friends becoming sexually active so I began to think it's all right. Well then you came along and definitely gave me a wakeup call." – Niki

Safer Sex

After reading thousands of letters from teenagers and young adults, it's obvious to me that many aren't practicing abstinence – the majority of them are sexually active. The CDC reports that teens are having their first sexual experiences at younger ages. Ask any middle school teacher about the sexual activity of 12 and 13-year-olds, and you'll be shocked at some of the stories.

Regardless of your age, if you're sexually active, or thinking about it, there are steps you can take to minimize your risk of contracting HIV or any other sexually transmitted disease.

If you're contemplating a sexual relationship with anyone, you should understand that whether or not you are legally an adult, sex is an adult activity and requires both partners to be mature enough to take responsibility for their actions. To avoid an unwanted pregnancy, contracting HIV or another sexually transmitted disease, you must learn to behave as an adult, even if you're not yet legally one. You must learn how to reduce your risks by having safer sex.

Notice I suggested you learn what needs to be done to have "safer sex." I did not use the term "safe sex." **There is no such thing as safe sex.** You can reduce the risk of an unwanted pregnancy or contracting STDs by having safer sex, but you cannot completely eliminate it.

There are precautions that single sexually-active individuals of any age can take to help minimize risk for not only themselves, but also their partners. Other adults often compliment me for the time and effort I spend talking with youth about HIV prevention. People often make comments such as, "*Don, it's great that you volunteer so much time to teach teenagers about HIV/AIDS. … Most teenagers have the attitude that, 'It can't happen to me.' … Young people are so careless and irresponsible, they need to hear what you have to say.*"

While it's true that teenagers are young, I've learned that being young does not automatically make someone careless. Over the years, I've met a number of teenagers who are more responsible and more "adult" in their sexual behavior than many people I know in their 30s, 40s and even older. Many who are older and dating don't feel the need to use condoms because they rely on the pill or some other form of birth control. Birth control pills are convenient, but they don't help prevent exposure to HIV or any other STD.

One of the fastest-growing rates of new HIV infection in the U.S. is in the retirement community. Here it's rare for anyone dating to use condoms. In fact, only six percent of those over the age of 60 use condoms on a fairly consistent basis. HIV does not discriminate. The risk of contracting HIV/AIDS exists for anyone of any age.

Here are four steps that single individuals **of all ages** can follow to help minimize the risks of contracting HIV/AIDS and other STDs:

1. **Assume everyone you are sexually involved with "might" be infected with HIV/AIDS**

2. **In the past, if you or your partner were sexually active with someone else, shared needles, syringes or drug paraphernalia, have an HIV test before engaging in any sexual activity**

3. **Have a discussion with your partner about the risks involved in various sexually activities and determine which activities are allowable**

4. **Always use a condom properly**

If you're not comfortable having an adult conversation with your potential partner to discuss these four points prior to having sex, I suggest you keep your clothes on. Failing to understand the risks involved, and setting up ground rules prior to sexual activity to help minimize them, can quite literally be deadly.

Step 1: Assume everyone might be HIV-positive

More than likely, you currently make the assumption whenever you go out with someone that he or she is not infected with HIV or any other STD. **Instead of automatically believing everyone you date is HIV-negative, I would encourage you to train yourself to assume anyone you're involved with "might" be infected with the virus.**

When you go to the dentist, what is the first thing he or she does before examining your teeth? The dentist puts on gloves. If there's a traffic accident, what is the first thing the police or paramedics do before touching someone who is injured? They put on gloves. Why the gloves? Because the dentist, the police and the paramedics want to avoid contact with anyone's blood. The primary reason that medical personnel wear gloves is because they have no idea if those they come in contact with have HIV/AIDS or some other blood-borne disease. **To be safe, they assume everyone they treat "might" be infected.**

When I was growing up, my dentist never wore gloves. He washed his hands and then put them in my mouth. Why no gloves? Because when I was a child, no one was aware HIV existed. Prior to HIV/AIDS, dentists assumed it was safe to put their bare hands into someone's mouth. Today, they know better. You'll be safer, and you'll reduce your risk of contracting HIV, if you start to think like your dentist.

Perhaps you think it's a bit extreme for me to suggest that you assume **everyone** you date **might** be infected with HIV/AIDS. After all, you know the person you are currently dating and you may be completely confident in assuming he or she doesn't have HIV. How-ever, do you know the sexual history of his or her previous sexual partners?

Sexual Exposure

When you have sex with someone, you're not just having sex with that one person. You're having sex with everyone they've had sex with over their lifetime, and everyone they and their partner(s) have had sex with during their lifetime.

The charts on the following two pages will help you better understand the definition and shocking consequences of having a high sexual exposure.

What Is Sexual Exposure?

When you have sex with someone, you're not just having sex with that one person. You are, in effect, having sex with everyone they've had sex with over their lifetime, and everyone their partners have had sex with during their lifetime.

If you and your partner are both virgins, and you have sex with each other, you each have had one sexual exposure.

Now assume that neither of you is a virgin and that you both have had sex with only one other person. Each of you now has a sexual exposure to three people: the two people you had sex with and the first person your partner had sex with.

Now assume that you've had sex with three different people. You're the first for your first partner, the second for your second partner and the third for your most recent partner. Each of you has been sexually exposed to seven different people.

The chart on the next page takes the same assumptions used in the above examples and expands the numbers.

What Is Your Sexual Exposure?

Number of previous sexual partners:	Total number of sexual exposures:
1	1
2	3
3	7
4	15
5	31
6	63
7	127
8	255
9	511
10	1,023
11	2,047
12	4,095
13	8,191
14	16,383
15	32,767
16	65,535
17	131,071
18	262,143
19	524,287
20	1,048,575

This simple model assumes everyone has had the same number of previous sexual partners.

This chart clearly illustrates the high risk of having multiple sex partners.

It's frightening, once you realize the implications of having multiple partners. Over the years, I've heard from thousands of teenagers with a history of more than one sexual partner. In most cases, he or she has had two or three previous partners, but it's common for high school students to reveal the fact they've already had six to 12 partners. On a number of occasions, I've been told, *"I really don't know how many people I've had sex with."*

Comments: Multiple Partners

"Dear Don Carrel ... The other thing that caught my attention was the fact that if you have had sex with 12 people, through the chains, you could indirectly have sex with 4,095 people." – *Tyler*

"Dear Don ... I will make sure my friend goes with me to see you. She is 16 years old and lost her virginity 3 months ago and has already been sexually active with 14 guys. I've tried to talk to her, but she thinks she is getting attention by this." – *Cheri*

"Don ... You made me realize a lot of things ... like sex isn't worth your life. I talked to my friend last night about everything you told us. I asked her how many people she's had sex with. She told me more than 20. Me, myself, I'm a proud virgin and plan to stay that way thanks to you." – *Anonymous*

Comments: Assuming everyone "might" be HIV-Positive

"Mr. Carrel looked good for someone with AIDS. That shows that when you meet a guy or girl, just because they look healthy doesn't mean anything. He said instead of assuming they aren't infected with HIV you should assume they are. I think those words will stick with me forever." – *Anonymous*

"Dear Don ... I have practiced risky behavior in the past but I always thought, oh, it happens, but not at East, not in Olathe, not with anyone I know. I think it hit me when you said you attended Shawnee Mission North and went to K-State. I realized HIV is now here, all around me. I've decided to practice abstinence from now on. Next Thursday me, and two of my best friends are going to be tested for HIV. I pray it's not too late. I'm really scared, but I can't ever thank you enough for making me realize what I'm doing." – *Anonymous*

"Hi Don ... The presentation gave me more of a 'wake up' signal. From your speech I have learned that anyone can get HIV easier than what people think. You taught me how to be more aware of what I do and to think differently. I will always remember what you said about dating and always have in mind that the person I am dating might have the disease and not know."
– Susan

"Don ... I thought the stories about your friends, Dennis and Kenny, were devastating. You helped me realize how careful I need to be in the future, and now, that I need to assume anyone I date or go out with could have AIDS. I wish you could do your presentation for the world." – Amanda

HIV/AIDS Disclosure

When I suggest you assume the person you're involved with "might" be HIV-positive, it's not because there are a lot of people with HIV/AIDS who conceal their status from their partners. The majority of those who are aware they have HIV share their positive status with potential partners. However, there are hundreds of thousands of Americans with HIV who aren't aware they're infected. Typically, a newly infected individual doesn't develop any symptoms of the disease for the first eight to 12 years that he or she is positive. Without taking the initiative to be tested to learn one's HIV status, it's quite possible for someone infected with the virus to spread it to others for years without being aware they're doing so.

Unfortunately, there are a small percentage of people who are aware they are HIV-positive do not inform their potential sex partners of their status.

If you have a history of multiple partners and/or typically engage in what might be called "one-night stands," there's a much greater chance that your partner of the moment will either be unaware of his or her status, or won't reveal that information to you.

If you're involved with someone who cares about you who happens to have HIV, he or she likely will inform you in advance of any sexual activity. However, if you're involved with someone who cares about you, but is unaware they're HIV-positive, he or she will not be able to inform you about your potential risk.

Step 2: Get tested for HIV

If there's even a slight risk you may have been exposed to HIV, there are two primary reasons I recommend you be tested for the virus. First, if you're HIV-positive, you want to be aware of your status so you can always take precautions to minimize the risk of infecting someone you care about. Second, if you're infected, you should consider starting medical treatment as soon as possible, before the virus has substantially compromised your immune system. Starting medical treatment early can help ensure that you live a longer, healthier life.

If you've had sex with someone whose history of sexual partners and/or drug use is unknown to you, or if you or your partner have had many sexual partners, then your chance of having HIV is higher than normal. **Both you and your new partner should be tested for HIV and learn the results before having sex the first time.**

If you're sexually active and unmarried, I recommend you and your partner be tested for HIV on a regular basis – preferably every six to 12 months. Always keep in mind that a "negative" HIV test result from a test taken today doesn't guarantee the person isn't infected with HIV. If the person who was tested today was infected within in the last six months, the test results may not be accurate.

Comments: HIV Testing

"Dear Don … Just this past month, a family friend of ours was exposed to HIV. She's currently 19 and had unprotected sex. Her partner called her about a month ago and told her that he has AIDS. She went to get tested immediately and she tested positive. It was her first time having sex and now her life has dramatically changed. Her parents took it pretty hard, and so did I. I couldn't believe it. She calls me when she's really depressed and I haven't quite known how to help her. But now thanks to you, I have a little bit more of an understanding or what she's going through, and unfortunately of what's to come." – Heather

Dear Don … I learned that you don't need parental permission to get tested (for HIV) which is great because that's probably 90% of the reason why kids don't get tested. If I was having underage premarital sex, I wouldn't tell my parents" – Whitney

Step 3: The risks of various sexual activities

Having sex is an adult activity, and I strongly recommend that two people contemplating a new sexual relationship sit down together and have a serious discussion prior to having sex. The conversation should include a discussion about the risks associated with various sexual activities and establish boundaries based on the amount of risk each is willing to take.

The reason sexual activity is a risk for HIV transmission is because it allows for the exchange of body fluids. Certain sexual practices are associated with a higher risk of transmission than others based on the likelihood body fluids will be exchanged.

Safer sex is not just about intercourse. There are a number of no-risk activities that don't result in the exchange of blood, semen or vaginal fluid. These activities include such things as hugging, kissing, cuddling, massage and masturbation. Younger couples, or even older couples in the beginning stages of their sexual relationship, may initially prefer to limit their activities to these types of safer behavior.

The question I get more than any other one is, ***"Can I get HIV from oral sex?"*** My response, *"Yes you can but the risk of contracting HIV from oral sex is much lower than the risk from intercourse."* The chance of contracting HIV from oral sex is relatively low, especially when compared to vaginal or anal intercourse. However, it's possible for either partner to become infected with HIV by performing or receiving oral sex. According to the CDC:

- There have been a few known cases of HIV transmission from performing oral sex on a person infected with HIV.

- If the person performing oral sex has HIV, blood from their mouth may enter the body of the person receiving oral sex through the lining of the urethra (the opening at the tip of the penis), the lining of the vagina or directly into the body through small cuts or open sores.

- If the person receiving oral sex has HIV, their blood, semen (cum), pre-seminal fluid (pre-cum) or vaginal fluid may contain the virus. If the person performing oral sex has cuts or sores around or in the mouth or throat, or bleeding gums, HIV may enter their body.

• The risk of HIV transmission via oral sex increases if the person receiving oral sex ejaculates in the mouth of the person performing oral sex; or if the person receiving oral sex has another sexually transmitted disease.

• To minimize the risk of HIV transmission while performing oral sex, use a latex condom if your partner is male. If your partner is female, use a latex barrier (such as a dental dam, a cut-open condom or plastic food wrap) between your mouth and the vagina. A barrier reduces the risk of blood or vaginal fluid entering your mouth.

When using a latex condom for oral sex, always use a non-lubricated condom. The lubricant on a regular condom tastes terrible and is not intended for ingestion.

Flavored condoms are available and are marketed as a way to improve the experience of performing safer oral sex. When purchasing flavored condoms, make sure they aren't labeled strictly as a novelty item. If you purchase flavored condoms from a well-known condom manufacturer, many of them are also FDA approved for strength and protection, and may be used safely for intercourse.

Even though the risk of transmission of HIV through oral sex is considered low, the transmission of other STDs through oral sex is very common.

Sexually transmitted diseases (STDs)

Genital Herpes

Genital herpes is an STD cause by viruses, either the HSV-1 or the HSV-2. According to the CDC, HSV-1 can cause genital herpes, but more commonly causes infections of the mouth or lips called "fever blisters."

HSV-1 is in the saliva and blood of people who carry the virus and is easily spread by direct exposure to saliva (kissing). HSV-1 infection of the genitals can be spread by oral-genital (oral sex), genital-genital or genital-anal contact with a person who has HSV-1 infection.

Genital HSV-2 occurs during the same sexual activities mentioned above with someone who has a genital HSV-2 infection.

According to the CDC, most individuals with genital herpes experience no symptoms or minimal signs of the disease. When symptoms do occur, they typically appear as one or more blisters on or around the genitals or rectum. The blisters break, leaving tender sores that normally heal within two to four weeks. Typically, another outbreak can appear weeks or months after the first, but it normally is less severe and shorter than the first outbreak.

Nationwide, about one of every six people between the ages of 14 and 49 have genital herpes. There is no cure for herpes, but treatment is available to reduce the symptoms and decrease the risk of transmission to a partner.

HPV (Human Papillomavirus)

HPV is the most common sexually-transmitted virus in the U.S. At least 50 percent of those who are sexually active will have genital HPV some time in their lives. HPV can cause genital warts on both males and females, and may lead to the development of cervical or anal cancer in the future.

HPV is easily transmitted via oral sex and it is believed that HPV transmitted during oral sex may be a major risk factor for throat cancer.

There is no cure for HPV. However, there is a vaccine to prevent HPV infection. **I recommend that all youth (both male and female) be vaccinated for HPV prior to becoming sexually active.**

Chlamydia

Chlamydia is the most frequently reported STD in the U.S. It is known as a "silent" disease because the majority of infected people have virtually no symptoms. If left untreated, chlamydia can damage a woman's reproductive system and possibly cause infertility. Chlamydia occasionally causes painful urination and/or a discharge from the penis of an infected man. Chlamydia can be easily treated and cured with antibiotics.

Chlamydia is easily transmitted during oral, vaginal or anal sex.

Gonorrhea

Gonorrhea, commonly called "clap," is the second most common infectious disease in the U.S. It's a bacterium that can grow in the cervix, uterus, urethra, mouth, throat and anus. It's easily treatable with antibiotics.

Both men and women can get gonorrhea. Some men with gonorrhea have no symptoms at all. However, most men have symptoms that appear two to five days (occasionally as long as 30 days) after the infection enters the urethra. Symptoms include a burning sensation when urinating, or a white, yellow, or green discharge from the penis. Most women who are infected have no symptoms. Rectal infections in men or women may cause no symptoms or can include discharge, anal itching, soreness, bleeding, or painful bowel movements.

Gonorrhea infections in the throat that result from oral sex may cause a sore throat, but usually have no symptoms. This STD is easily transmitted to either partner during oral, vaginal or anal sex.

"Non-Specific" Urethritis (NGU)

NGU is an infection of the urethra (the tube that carries urine through the body in both men and women) caused by germs other than **gonorrhea**. Antibiotics are used to treat NGU.

Symptoms for men and women include penile or vaginal discharge, burning while urinating or itching. NGU can lead to significant health problems including infertility in men, and chronic pelvic pain and pelvic inflammatory disease (PID) in women.

NGU can be transmitted through oral, vaginal or anal sex, even if body fluids do not appear to be exchanged and there is no "total" penetration.

Syphilis

Syphilis can be transmitted during vaginal, anal or oral sex.

Syphilis is caused by a bacterium and is passed from person to person through direct contact with a syphilis sore called a chancre. Chancres occur mainly on the external genitals, vagina, anus, or in the rectum, but they can also occur on the lips and in the mouth.

Many people infected with syphilis don't have symptoms for many years. Although transmission occurs from contact with chancres, many of these sores aren't recognized as syphilis because people often assume they're something as minor as a pimple. The time between infection with syphilis and the first symptom can range from 10 to 90 days (average 21 days). A small chancre appears at the spot where the disease entered the body. The sore goes away without treatment. A single injection of penicillin, or other antibiotics, will normally cure a person who has had the disease for less than a year.

Syphilis has often been called "the great imitator" because so many of the signs and symptoms are indistinguishable from those of other diseases. During late stages, the disease can cause blindness, paralysis, dementia and death.

Hepatitis B (HBV)

Hepatitis B is irritation and inflammation of the liver. HBV is spread through contact with body fluids, including blood, vaginal fluids and semen. Symptoms of HBV can include fever, loss of appetite, vomiting, abdominal pain, nausea, dark urine, jaundice (yellow skin or eyes) and muscle or joint pain.

Research concerning Hepatitis B and transmission via oral sex is not conclusive. However, oral-anal contact can definitely transmit the Hepatitis B virus.

There are no specific medications to cure acute Hepatitis B. However, even without treatment, most people recover completely within a few months.

You can protect yourself from Hepatitis B by having a vaccination to prevent infection from the virus.

Hepatitis A (HAV)

Hepatitis A is a virus that also results in irritation and swelling of the liver. It is found in the stool of people with the Hepatitis A virus. It's usually spread through close personal contact, such as shaking hands with or eating food prepared by someone with the virus who failed to wash their hands after using the restroom.

While not normally considered to be an STD, Hepatitis A can be spread by oral-anal contact with an infected person.

As with Hepatitis B, you can be vaccinated against Hepatitis A to prevent infection from the virus.

Hepatitis C (HCV)

Hepatitis C is a contagious, viral disease and like Hepatitis A and B, it leads to swelling of the liver. HCV can range in severity from a mild illness lasting a few weeks to a serious, lifelong illness.

Most people who are infected with HCV develop chronic liver problems that can result in long-term health problems, and even death. Like HIV, Hepatitis C is spread when blood from a person who is infected gets into the bloodstream of someone who is not infected. Most of those who contract HCV do so by sharing needles to inject drugs.

HCV is rarely detected in semen and vaginal fluids and as a result, most experts believe the risk of sexual transmission of HCV is low.

There is no vaccine for Hepatitis C.

There is no doubt that unprotected oral sex puts you at risk for many sexually transmitted diseases. If you perform unprotected oral sex and an STD infection occurs in your throat, there are rarely any symptoms. If oral sex is an activity you participate in, tell your physician, so she or he can check your throat when screening you for STDs.

Many adolescents who engage in oral sex don't consider it "real" sex. Therefore, they may view oral sex as an option to experience sex, but in their minds believe they're remaining abstinent. Oral sex is definitely "real" sex when you consider it carries a high risk of contracting sexually transmitted diseases.

Comments: Oral Sex

"Hi Don ... I'm scared because I never knew that you could catch AIDS from oral sex. The point is that it's a good thing that I'm scared because it means you're getting the message across. Yesterday when I left that room, I realized that everything you said made sense. Sex is a powerful weapon and if you abuse it and don't save it for the person you love, then it can hurt you, or even literally kill you. I wish I could take back some things in my past concerning the sex issue, but I can't. The only thing that I can do is take precautions, so that I try to remain abstinent in the near future. You've reached me and gotten the message across, and Don, let me tell you a little something ... I'm the most stubborn person on the face of the earth. ... You'll be in my thoughts and prayers." – Andrew

"Dear Don ... You have probably saved me from getting AIDS. I got at least 50 blow jobs last summer and had sex a couple of times with protection and a couple of times unprotected. I'm going to get tested next time I'm in Westport because the place you told us about looks like it's close to there. Your presentation also saved me from potentially using dirty needles. I'm not going to lie to you. I smoke weed almost every day and I've done OxyContin a couple of times and everyone says it's a lot

better when you shoot it up. I'm not going to mess around from here on out because of what you said about moving up the drug ladder. The drug ladder is true and it's bad news. I just wanted you to know that you potentially saved my life." – Jake

Engaging in oral sex, while much less risky than having vaginal or anal intercourse, is not risk free. There are several co-factors that increase the likelihood of contracting HIV through oral sex, including cold sores, genital sores, bleeding gums (do not floss or brush your teeth prior to performing oral sex), oral ulcers, having other STDs or allowing someone to ejaculate in your mouth.

Step 4: Always "properly" use a condom

Hopefully, by this point, you understand the reasons and importance of going through the previous three steps. By assuming your partner "might" have HIV, being tested for HIV if needed and discussing which sexual activities and risks are acceptable, you'll have accomplished a great deal of what is necessary to help prevent you from contracting HIV.

I know it might appear to be unromantic and far too formal to have such a conversation, but considering the possible consequences, it's worth the inconvenience and any embarrassment to do so. If you're not comfortable, willing or ready to have an adult conversation with your partner about completing these steps, I highly recommend you keep your clothes on. This recommendation applies to everyone, regardless of age.

If you've completed the first three steps, you are ready for Step 4: Always "Properly" Use a Condom.

In today's world of HIV/AIDS, it's important that you view a condom primarily as a "disease prevention tool" and not a birth control device. In addition to condoms, there are pills and other forms of birth control available for use to help avoid pregnancy. However, other than abstinence, there's no device that is effective in preventing HIV other than a condom. For those of you of the Catholic faith who follow strict church doctrine and don't believe in using condoms, keep in mind that if you're sexually active outside of a committed, marital relationship, you're at a much higher risk of infection for HIV and other STDs than those who understand the necessity of using condoms.

According to the CDC, someone having anal or vaginal intercourse without a condom with a partner who is positive, or isn't aware of his or her HIV status, accounts for the vast majority of sexually transmitted HIV cases in the U.S.

Unprotected anal sex is the riskiest of all forms of sexual intercourse. Mentioning anal intercourse is often considered taboo, especially when discussed in the context of teenage relationships. However, anal sex is more prevalent with teenagers and young adults than one might think, and it is a significant risk factor for not only HIV, but also other STDs:

- A CDC survey in 2008 found that 16 percent of teens and young adults between the ages of 15 and 21 had engaged in anal sex at least once in the previous three months

- Studies have shown that teenagers who take virginity/abstinence pledges are more likely to engage in anal sex than non-pledging teens because they don't consider it "real" sex

The incidence of anal sex is on the rise among teenagers and young adults. There are many reasons teenagers and young adults often engage in anal sex:

- Anal sex eliminates the possibility of pregnancy

- Many younger people don't consider anal sex to be "real" sex and as a result believe that having it does not rob them of their virginity

- Most younger people mistakenly believe they cannot get HIV or other STDs from anal sex

- Some agree to have anal intercourse to please their partner who has expressed an interest in it

- Anal sex is sometimes a substitution for vaginal intercourse when a condom is not readily available

It's critical that we recognize more young people are engaging in anal sex and that we open the lines of communications between teens, parents and health care providers on the subject. That open dialogue between health care providers and their young patients about anal intercourse is paramount. Clinicians should ask about anal sex during discussions about vaginal intercourse and protection regardless of the patient's gender or purported sexual orientation.

Studies have shown that if condoms are used **properly and consistently** every time you have sex, they're 98 percent effective in preventing pregnancy. The CDC reports that condoms are very effective in preventing HIV infection. In a two-year study of couples where one partner was HIV-positive and the other HIV-negative, no HIV-negative partner was infected when condoms were used correctly and consistently during every sexual encounter. Among the couples where condom use was inconsistent, 10 percent of the HIV-negative partners became infected during the two years.

Consistent and proper use of condoms dramatically reduces the risk of pregnancy and HIV infection. Condoms also reduce the risk for many STDs transmitted by genital fluids and diseases such as chlamydia and gonorrhea. In addition, the risk of contracting genital herpes, syphilis, genital human papillomavirus (HPV) infection and HPV-associated diseases (e.g., genital warts and cervical cancer) are also reduced with the use of condoms.

A number of years ago, I gave a presentation to a group of about 50 students at Avila University in Kansas City, Missouri. Avila has a number of programs that attract older students, and most of those who heard me that day were 35 and older. It was a more mature, sexually experienced crowd than I typically encounter. Those attending were comfortable asking specific questions regarding safer sex. I asked the group a few questions about proper use of condoms and it became apparent that not one of the 50 adults in attendance knew how to use a condom correctly.

Using a condom "consistently" requires you to use one **every** time you have vaginal or anal intercourse. Here's what I think you must do to use a condom **properly**:

- Learn to put a condom on correctly. If the condom does not have a reservoir tip, pinch the tip enough to leave a half-inch of space for semen to collect. If you put on a condom and don't leave some space at the tip, you increase the likelihood the condom will break.

- Always use condoms that are in good condition. Condoms will deteriorate if not stored properly and their quality can be affected by heat, light and age.

- Condom packages are marked with expiration dates. Always use condoms that have not yet reached the expiration date.

- Never re-use a condom. Use a new condom for every act of vaginal, anal and oral sex.

- Ensure that adequate lubrication is used during vaginal and anal sex and **always use a water-based lubricant with a latex condom.** Oil-based lubricants (e.g., petroleum jelly, mineral oil, massage oils, baby oil, body lotions, vegetable oil or shortening) should not be used because they can weaken a latex condom, causing breakage.

- If you're allergic to latex and cannot use a latex condom, use a condom made of polyurethane. Polyurethane condoms are thinner than latex condoms and some people actually prefer them as they may increase sensitivity.

- There are also condoms made of "natural" materials such as lambskin. Lambskin condoms are not effective as a barrier against HIV. They contain microscopic holes that may permit the virus to penetrate.

- If you notice a condom break at any point during sexual activity, stop immediately, withdraw, remove the broken condom and put on a new one.

- Never wear two condoms (called "double bagging") at the same time. It may seem that wearing two condoms is better than one, since the extra condom would protect you if one condom broke. However, double bagging causes friction between the two condoms making it easier for both to break during intercourse.

- Another precaution you can take to further reduce the risk if your condom should break or leak during use is **to withdraw from your partner before ejaculation.** By doing so, you significantly reduce the risk your semen will come into contact with your partner's body fluids.

I've always stressed the last point – about withdrawing from your partner **before ejaculation** – because common sense indicates it would maximize protection. While writing this book, I researched for other suggestions about the proper use of condoms. I was surprised to learn that the CDC guidelines on how to use a condom "consistently and correctly" did not include withdrawal before ejaculation. Instead, the CDC recommends that "After ejaculating and before the penis gets soft, grip the rim of the condom and carefully withdraw. Then gently pull the condom off, making sure that semen does not spill out."

According to the CDC, if you consistently use a condom in good condition and use it correctly, there's less than a 2 percent chance you'll contract HIV or end up with an unwanted pregnancy. This 2 percent chance of infection or pregnancy is based on the CDC's guidelines for condom use. My point is that it only makes sense that if you withdraw from your partner before ejaculation, your risk will be even smaller.

A number of years ago, I was giving a presentation to a group of about 300 students taking health at a local high school. After I was finished, there was time for questions and one of the teenage males in the audience raised his hand and said, ***"I always use a condom, but most of the time it breaks during sex."*** I responded by saying, *"That is really odd, because I'm almost 50 years old, and I've <u>never</u> had a condom break."* In the course of trying to figure out why this young man's condoms were always breaking, I asked, *"Where do you keep your condoms?"* His response, *"I hide them in a little box under the front seat of my car. I can't take them in the house, because I'm afraid my parents will find them."*

Condom packages are stamped with expiration dates for a good reason. They should also be stamped with a warning that says, *"Please keep me at room temperature."*

The plain and simple fact is that condoms deteriorate when exposed to heat, which dramatically increases the chance of breakage. On a summer day, the temperature inside a closed vehicle can reach 40 degrees above the outside temperature in less than an hour. If you store condoms in your car and roll up the windows, it won't take long for the heat to weaken the latex to the point they're likely to break during use. I've repeated the "condoms in the car" story to thousands of teenagers since I first heard it. Many of them have confessed that they, too, kept condoms in their cars.

It might also be a good idea to stamp another warning on condoms, *"Please don't sit on me."* When I was in high school, like many of my friends, I carried a condom in my wallet for months at a time just in case I might get "lucky" and happen to need one. Thankfully, I never got lucky. After sitting on my wallet and condom for months, I'm sure it wasn't in usable condition when I finally tossed it in the trash. If you conducted a survey of all the men in the U.S., I have no doubt that millions of them would admit that they at one time had a condom tucked away in their wallet.

Condoms and Teenagers

Discussing the word "condoms" and "teenagers" in the same sentence is often a subject of great debate. Should teens be given ready access to condoms and be told how to use them correctly? Or does educating teens about condom use encourage them to engage in sex? It's a fact that all teens will not abstain from sex. It's also a fact that condoms are effective in reducing teen pregnancy, the spread of HIV and other STDs.

I have two sons, Chris and Matt, who were once teenagers. As their father, I preferred that they refrained from sex while they were teenagers and told them so. However, I also made it clear that if they were going to have sex and were too embarrassed to purchase their own condoms, I would buy them. What was my alternative? I definitely didn't want either of my sons to become a teenage father, or worse, a teenager with HIV.

When parents are open and honest about the use of condoms with their teenagers, they're three times more likely to use condoms. The teens also are less likely to end up pregnant or with an STD. However, it's vital that parents discuss condom use early, **before** their teen has his or her first sexual encounter.

To their credit, teenagers as a whole do a much better job of consistently using condoms than their elders. A recent study of more than 3,400 people who agreed it was important to always use a condom revealed the following:

- Those ages 14 to 17 used a condom 68 percent of the time
- Those ages 18 to 24 used a condom 42 percent of the time
- Those ages 25 to 34 used a condom 27 percent of the time
- Those ages 35 to 44 used a condom 14 percent of the time
- Those ages 45 to 60 used a condom 12 percent of the time
- Those 61 and older used a condom 6.5 percent of the time

A condom's effectiveness largely depends on the person using it. Occasionally, I hear what I consider to be misleading statistics about condoms having high failure rates. Failure rates can be significant if you don't use a condom in good condition, consistently and correctly. However, failure rates are low if you follow the steps discussed in this chapter regarding their use.

I also have heard on more than one occasion the rumor that the HIV virus is small enough to pass through a condom and therefore, condoms aren't effective in preventing HIV infection. However, according to the CDC, "Laboratory studies have demonstrated that latex condoms provide an essentially impermeable barrier to particles the size of HIV."

If you consistently use a condom that is in good condition and always use it properly, there is less than a two percent chance you will contract HIV or end up with an unwanted pregnancy.

Comments: Condoms

"I am very thankful Don came to talk. I don't think he will ever understand just how much he helped others and me. He is truly a blessing from God. One of the most important things that I got from Don's presentation is that if you can't have a mature conversation with your partner about having safe sex and using a condom every time then you aren't ready for sex. I think that was a very good message." – Arianna

"Hi Don ... I know <u>now</u> how important it is to have safer sex. I have only had one sex partner and we still have sex. We have never been tested. I think we will do that. I have had one condom break on me because I had it in my wallet." – David

"Don ... I would like to thank you, as extremely silly and weird as this sounds, for the info on proper use of a condom. Parents and teachers always tell us to use them, but not how. As I am female and worrying about STDs and pregnancy is a major issue. I won't be having sex anytime soon ... knowledge is power ... I have decided it is going to be a pre-requirement for my boyfriend and I to be tested should we decide to do something on the sexual level." – Megan

"Dear Don ... I learned a lot today. One thing I thought was very interesting is to never keep a condom in a wallet. Most guys I know usually do that to look cool, but hopefully now they know how dangerous that can be." – Venny

"Dear Don ... I had a cousin and an uncle who died from AIDS and I know how painful it can be for you to lose someone. I'm really glad that my mom took time to sit down with me and talk about AIDS and she told me that if I do have sex that I should use protection. A lot of my friends, their parents, don't take time to talk with them because they just assume that their child isn't having sex, so they don't use protection. I went back and

told all my friends that they need to use protection or don't have sex at all. I'd hate to see them get HIV." – Andrea

"Hi Don ... I thought it was great that you talked about the fact a lot of people don't know they are infected and that the use of condoms is not 100% protection. Most speakers wouldn't have talked about how to use a condom correctly and that's the only way to get 98 percent protection. ... I thought it was also a good thing you mentioned that if you find out you're HIV-positive you should call people you've slept with so they can get tested." – Jessica

"Dear Don ... I know that next year when I am at college I will party and probably have sex. I will try every time to use a condom. I want to be safe because I have so much going for me. Sex might be good, but it's not worth dying for." – Ryan

"Dear Mr. Carrel ... I'm not sexually active or anything like that, but I was born with some strange problem that does not allow me to have children so I was never going to wear a condom. You have convinced me otherwise, so I will wear one to protect myself from HIV and STDs." – Nate

"Dear Don ... Well a little about myself. I will be turning 15 in three days. I don't plan on having sex, until I marry. ... Some people don't want to go to the store and look for condoms and buy them. For a present I plan to get some of my friends condoms. They will think it's a joke but it won't be. I don't want my friends to get pregnant or to get a nasty disease." – Laura

Dear Don ... Your presentation <u>*really hit home!*</u> *I never really paid attention to AIDS before you talked to us. Whenever my friends think about taking their clothes off I always tell them to wrap it." – Kallen*

Alcohol, drugs and HIV

It's a fact; the use of alcohol or drugs increases the risk you'll be infected with HIV. Obviously, if you choose to have one beer or a hit of weed, you're not going to contract the virus from the beer or the weed. However, the more alcohol you consume and/or the more illegal drugs you put into your system, the more likely you'll end up intoxicated or high enough that your behavior will put you at risk for HIV. Those under the influence of drugs and/or alcohol do careless, stupid and dangerous things.

I first realized just how significant the use of alcohol and drugs were in increasing the risk of HIV infection a number of years ago while volunteering as an HIV testing counselor. Once I began meeting with people who came into the clinic for an HIV test, I soon learned that the majority of them came because they had done something careless after drinking or doing drugs.

The following is a true story that explains how someone who might not normally be at risk for HIV/AIDS can quickly put himself or herself in danger while under the influence of alcohol.

The Kansas City Free Health Clinic in Kansas City, Missouri, provides basic health care services at no charge to people who cannot afford care and are without health insurance. Most of the individuals who rely on KC Free are poor, and sometimes homeless. In addition to providing excellent health care, the clinic offers free HIV testing. I frequently recommend KC Free as a place for anyone, including teenagers, to be tested for HIV because those who volunteer at the clinic are trained to help make anyone who comes for an HIV test feel comfortable during the process.

One morning, as soon as the clinic opened, a man who appeared to be about 35 walked in and quietly inquired about having an HIV test. After learning the clinic's HIV testing didn't start for another hour, he settled into a chair in the waiting room. The man fidgeted nervously in his seat, frequently checked his watch and seemed to be quite apprehensive. I couldn't help but notice the way he was dressed. His suit appeared to be custom-made and fit him perfectly. His shoes were polished, his nails flawlessly manicured and his jet-black hair professionally styled. He definitely wasn't typical of the patients who routinely rely upon a free clinic for their health care.

When HIV testing started that morning, I escorted this man – I'll call him "Brad" – into a small office, not much larger than a closet. I asked Brad if there was any particular event that had occurred to make him believe he needed an HIV test, or did he just come in to have a routine test to check his status?

Brad told me that he was a lawyer who had just returned from spending four days in New Orleans. He went with a small group from his office to attend a two-day business meeting and then spent the weekend relaxing in New Orleans. On Saturday night, Brad and a couple of his co-workers decided to go the French Quarter for dinner and drinks. He ended up drinking more than normal. In fact, Brad ended up drunk – so drunk that he hired a prostitute. When Brad woke up sober on Sunday morning, he realized how careless he had been. **While he was drunk, he had intercourse with a prostitute, and he did not use a condom.**

Brad did indeed have good reason to worry. Prostitutes typically have 200 to 300 sexual partners per year. With such an unusually high number of partners, those selling sex have a much higher exposure risk to HIV than average. In addition, prostitutes have a high rate of intravenous drug use, which also puts them at a higher risk for HIV infection.

I also learned that even though Brad was not married, he had been involved in a monogamous relationship for the past five years. His girlfriend was taking birth control pills, so they never used condoms.

When Brad finished explaining why he "urgently" needed to be tested for HIV, I had to tell him what I'm sure he considered bad news. I explained that if he had been exposed to HIV on Saturday night during a one-night stand with a prostitute, it wouldn't show up on a test taken just two days after the encounter. I suggested he return to the clinic in six weeks for an HIV test. I also explained that if he tested negative in six weeks, the chances would be good that he wasn't infected with HIV. However, to be 100 percent certain he didn't contract HIV from the prostitute, he would need to come back for a follow-up test six months after the sexual encounter took place.

I let Brad know that if he did contract HIV on Saturday night, it was definitely possible for him to transmit the virus to his girlfriend before his positive status showed up on an HIV test. I suggested that he either abstain for the next six months until he received his follow-up test results, or to use a condom every time he had intercourse during the next six months. Brad turned white as a ghost, looked at me wide-eyed and said, *"How in the world am I going to tell my girlfriend we need to use condoms, when we haven't used them in five years?"*

Unfortunately, there was nothing I could say to help make the situation easier for Brad. I remember thinking at the time; *"I'm sure glad that the task of talking to Brad's girlfriend, and explaining why they needed to use condoms, was his problem and not mine."*

Since the day I met Brad at the Kansas City Free Health Clinic, I've told his story hundreds of times whenever I try to illustrate the connection between alcohol and the risk of contracting HIV. His is a good example for a couple of reasons. First, it clearly shows how excessive drinking can suddenly put someone not normally at risk for HIV into a high-risk situation. Second, it illustrates how a normally responsible adult put not only his life, but also his relationship in jeopardy, simply because he drank too much alcohol.

Brad was an adult, and more than likely had previous experience consuming alcohol. He should have known better. He should have already learned that people who are under the influence behave differently than those who are sober. They make poor, careless and flat-out stupid decisions that can put not only themselves, but also others in danger.

There is a valuable lesson to be learned from Brad's mistake.

Chris's story

About five years ago I met a trim, fit, intelligent young man named Chris. Chris was the receptionist and office assistant for my dentist. At the time I met Chris, he was just starting college at the University of Missouri–Kansas City and was planning to go to dental school after graduating. Chris's life took a drastic turn during his first year of college, when he started down the road of alcohol and drug abuse.

In the course of a year, Chris flunked out of UMKC. He was addicted to methamphetamines and tested positive for HIV. Here is his story in his words.

The teenage years are probably the hardest years of a person's life, as they try to find themselves. It's common for teens not to listen to adults, letting what they hear go in one ear and out the other without regard to importance.

I believe it's far too easy for young people to venture down the wrong path. My parents loved me and showed me that they loved me. However, both my mother and father worked a lot of overtime. When they were not working, they seemed to be distracted by something. Even when my parents were home, I didn't feel as if they were "fully present" ... we didn't really communicate ... we did not have a real relationship. It was because of this lack of parental attention that I searched to fulfill the need to feel important outside the home.

My self-esteem and self-image were shattered, causing me to think of myself as having little to no value. Feeling unimportant, I believed it was not necessary for me to listen or take to heart the warnings and lessons from my elders regarding drugs and unsafe sex.

For me, it was the pressure of feeling I would ultimately fail, which allowed me to slip easily into a destructive lifestyle of alcohol, drugs and unsafe sex. I set myself up for failure by thinking I had to conform and become the person my parents, teachers and friends wanted me to be. Struggling to succeed in the conformation, I found myself getting frustrated and acting out, because I wasn't sure who I was, nor did I seem to be succeeding in being who others wanted me to be. Wounded by my failure, I was vulnerable to negative outside influences.

At the tender age of 23, I stumbled upon a natural attraction to methamphetamines. My love for the drug grew considerably from August through the end of the year. It happened so quickly; I never knew what hit me. I was in my first semester at UMKC. By the end of the year, I had flunked out of school and on December 26, the day after Christmas, I found out from my doctor that I had tested positive for HIV.

At first, I thought I was properly dealing with the news of being HIV-positive. However, unbeknownst to me, I was slipping into a deep depression. With a negative outlook on life, I felt like I had nothing to live for. My desire to feel good led to a life of partying at bars and doing meth. Over the next year or so, my craving and subsequent use of meth became a part of daily life. My desire for meth was stronger than any friendship. My dealer eventually became my only friend, aside from meth. I was addicted to methamphetamines, and I knew it.

I wish my diagnosis had been enough for me to realize that I was headed down a very negative path. But I was heavily addicted to meth. I required the drug daily. I couldn't and wouldn't get out of bed without it. My use was not fueled by the desire to use; it was actually the opposite. I hated the drug and what I had become. I would use meth to get up in the morning and once or twice during the day. This was my daily ritual without fail. My drug dealer was the only person who remained in my life. He was the only person I wanted to see. And I did see him. I called him religiously. Almost like clockwork, once a week, we met so that I could restock for the week ahead. And sometimes I would call him once during the week when I ran out of meth.

I was spending between $125 and $250 every week on the drug. Money was never an issue. I had a very good job in construction, earning a great salary. Even when money was tight, due to the weather causing my weekly pay to be less than normal, I willingly gave up the money and was happy to do so. But the drug always wore off. Life was a continual cycle of highs and lows, peaks and valleys. I was never at peace with myself. I felt lost.

Once I was lost, it was easy for me to find all the wrong people to spend my free time with. At this point, I found myself searching for happiness through the use of alcohol, drugs and sex. I spent the majority of my time arranging my next drink, hit or looking for sex.

My general lack of desire to live turned into a desire to die. By this point, my daily meth use had taken its toll on my immune system. I was constantly sick with flu-like symptoms, and I lacked the energy to even get out of bed. Feeling like death was close, with my mother constantly pleading with me to seek medical help, I finally went to my doctor to see what was going on with my body. I went to the doctor mostly because I was sick of hearing my mother's whining and begging all the time, not because I was really concerned for my own well-being or scared that I was dying. In fact, I hoped I was dying.

My doctor expressed her concern stating "Chris, if you don't do something quick, you're going to be dead!" Finally, I was almost there. I was almost finished with this lifetime of suffering. Preparing myself for the end, I began thinking about all that I had experienced in my short life. I thought about the places I had been and the many places I had not yet been. I thought about my family, about my niece and nephew.

Maybe getting HIV was fate, working to slow me down and pull me back to my true nature. At the time I was first infected, I was living a very wild life, consumed by drugs and sex, with no regard for anything or anyone, including myself. Ironically, in many ways, I'm grateful for getting HIV. Without it, I could have lived my entire life with the same negative focus that was destroying me. However, the virus, in combination with my heavy drug use, quickly worked to weaken my immune system to the point that I was deathly ill, forcing me to review my life up to that point and helping me realize what is truly important in life.

In retrospect, I wish it wouldn't have taken such a drastic situation to occur before I came to this realization, since I'm forever more forced to live with the poor choices I've made. In most cases, people are given the opportunity to make right the poor choices they've made. However, I'm forced to live with my choices. No matter how I change my life for the better, I will forever more be an HIV-infected drug addict.

The adage, "it is not until something is lost, that its true importance is known," rings truer than ever to my ears. For it was not until I was literally almost dead that I realized life was important and worth living. It was not until I was heavily addicted to drugs that I realized they were not helping my life, but rather hindering it. It was not until I was HIV-positive that I realized unsafe sexual practices can be harmful.

Rather than dwelling on the past and feeling sorry for myself, I feel like I need to make something positive of my situation. I know that my life experiences in the last five years have been more dramatic than most people encounter in an entire lifetime. If sharing my experiences with sex and drugs with others can prevent them from having to find out for themselves, then I would feel an overwhelming sense of joy and fulfillment.

In 2010, Chris turned 28 and found relief from addiction and a new way of life since joining Narcotics Anonymous. Like many of those who have developed an alcohol and/or drug problem, Chris started down what seemed to be a safe path. He started with an occasional drink or two and occasionally smoked a little weed. Those initial steps into the world of alcohol and drugs led him down the path in search of bigger and better highs. Where did the path take Chris? His own words say it best, *"I will forever more be an HIV-infected drug addict."*

As a drug addict, Chris knows he must never again have even one beer or smoke any weed. Doing so would put him right back on the path to self-destruction. I'm so thankful Chris shared his life-shattering journey as a part of this book. His heartfelt story does a much better job of explaining how alcohol and drugs increase your risk for HIV infection than I ever could.

Chris believes it's vital that parents understand the importance of being *"fully present"* when they're with their children and working diligently to establish a close relationship with them early in their lives. He believes, *"You only get one chance to be a parent to your children. Once that time has passed, little you do to try to make up for lost time will matter."*

The following stories are from just a few of the teenagers I've had the privilege to share my story with over the years. By the time you finish reading their comments, hopefully, the connection between alcohol, drugs and HIV, will be crystal clear.

Comments: Alcohol, drugs & HIV/AIDS

"Dear Don ... I would like to thank you for speaking to my class. Some of the people in my class need a good scaring. Your really scared me when you talked about your friends and the trauma they went through. I was on the verge of tears when you were talking because I was worried and scared about my health.

About two weeks ago, at Spirit Fest, I was tripping, high and extremely drunk. Some girls I knew were helping me walk and they were slapping my face trying to keep me awake because I was passing out every second. I can't remember much of that night, but what I remember is so embarrassing. I remember trying to walk, and kissing every guy that held my hand or tried to hold me up. I was so drunk I even gave a guy a hand job in the middle of a big crowd. A lot of people from my school were there and saw me taking off my shirt and running around. I was so stupid.

On Tuesday when school started again, rumors were flying around that I had sex with everyone. Guys were telling people that I did stuff with them. I was mortified and scared to death. I don't remember half of the night, so pretty much anything is possible. Before I went to Spirit Fest I was a virgin and planned to stay like that until marriage. Those guys could have gotten me pregnant or given me some kind of disease. I just took a pregnancy test and I am going to wait two weeks and take another one. My best friend's boyfriend is going to drive me to a clinic to get tested for HIV. I never imagined myself a mother or a carrier of HIV/AIDS at the age of 14. My birthday was just two months ago. I'm young and was so stupid." – Love, Casey

"Dear Don ... My name is Grant and I'm in the 10th grade. Six months ago, I had sex with a prostitute and unfortunately, due to the fact that I had too much to drink that night, I made a fool-ish decision not to wear a condom.

To make sure I was okay, I went to get a blood test a week ago. The test took about 3 hours and going to the doctor for the test was the most embarrassing situation I have ever been in.

Right now as we speak, I have no clue as to what the results are, but I'm hoping for the best. Right now I don't know what to think, feel or do. Basically, I'm numb and worry about it everyday. I don't regret having sex; I just regret not wearing a condom. I appreciate the fact that you came to talk to us. For those who have not had sex, I think it was an eye opener. For those of us who have had sex, it was a reminder." – Grant

"Don ... Most of my friends have already had sex and go to parties, get wasted and have unprotected sex. I get angry at their choices, never them. I told my friends about you and they had some concern about themselves. That day I took 5 of them to the clinic you suggested. I'm proud to have done that. The results came in and none of them have HIV. Thanks to you I feel like I have saved my friends from getting AIDS." – Chelsea

"Dear Don ... I have some friends who I know that like to go to parties and drink and have sex with whoever they can find. What you are doing helped me realize how important the decisions I make are and that I should tell my friends to be careful when they're out messing around." – Matt

Dear Don ... I was just thinking today that just a little slip and I could be taking my own life. I drink a lot and with people that I don't really know that well. I know I get as careless as can be and think 'oh, that could never happen to me, or none of these people could possibly have this disease' I was just like 'whoa Kristen, you're not being smart about this at all.' ... I know for a fact that now I am going to watch myself and my actions." – Kristen

"Dear Don ... In your presentation I learned many important things. The most important thing I learned is how much the choices I make in having sex or doing anything else that can transmit AIDS determines the rest of my life. Every time I get drunk, I make bad choices and one of those choices is getting drunk in the first place. But one bad choice I make could easily give me AIDS, which would destroy my life." – Eric

"Dear Don ... In the past, I have been told to stay sex free and not to use IV drugs, but it all made sense when you said it. Just being educated about it is different than being given a real life example. ... I am very glad that at this point in my life I am 100% safe from HIV. Your speech stirred up a lot of emotions and made me think about life and my choices. I have nothing but respect for you, because I feel that you have reached your full potential in life. Not many people can say that. Thank you for making me a smarter and better person." – Dina

"Dear Don ... I am one of those people who always thought that it couldn't happen to me. I now understand that it can. My older brother got drunk one time and decided that for fun he and this other girl would have sex. Well apparently two other girls joined in. He found out later that one of the girls has AIDS. Luckily, my brother didn't get it, because he was smart enough to use a condom. My brother used a condom because he had heard you talk a couple of years ago. THANK YOU." – Love, Madison

"Don ... My thoughts about the AIDS virus are that I don't know a whole lot about it and my ignorance could be detrimental to my health. In Kansas City, MO, I know 6 people who have the disease. All of them are hetero, white males. I don't judge anyone with AIDS. I take risks also and I know that I'm not invincible and that I can <u>catch</u> it. ... I could have AIDS. I've been very careless over the summer. I'm scared and I've been told that one of the girls I was with could very well have the disease. I'm scared to go into the clinic. I definitely support your idea that drugs and alcohol increase the chance of people catching HIV. I was under the influence of illegal drugs when I chose to get careless and not use a rubber. Hopefully, I don't have anything. This weekend I'll get tested." – William

Intravenous drug use

Ask almost anyone with a history of intravenous drugs and he or she will tell you they didn't start their drug use with a needle. Most IV drug users started with a bit of marijuana or another less dangerous drug. However, the desire for a better high leads many drug users down the path to IV drugs, which can easily result in a drug overdose or a life of HIV/AIDS.

Sadly, those who contract HIV through IV drug use continue to spread the disease not only to their future drug partners, but also to their loved ones through sexual activity.

Having a healthy, satisfying sexual relationship with someone during our life is a desire most of us will strive to obtain. It's considered normal to want someone special in your life. In today's world, having a sexual relationship has risks, most of which can be avoided.

However, the use of intravenous drugs isn't a normal or expected part of life and those participating in this activity put themselves at great risk of living life with HIV/AIDS. If you make the decision to use intravenous drugs, it's not a question of *"Will you get HIV?"* – It's simply a question of – *"How soon will you have it?"* You can dramatically reduce your risk of ever contracting HIV/AIDS simply by making the decision to never use any drug that could start you down the path toward the use of intravenous drugs.

Comments: IV Drug Use

"Don … As far as my personal story … I do have one … about a year ago, I learned that my father was HIV positive. This news really scared me not only because my father might die, but because I could be infected, too.

My dad started taking drugs when I was two years old. He did heroin and other drugs intravenously. This is how I believe he contracted the virus. There were people at our house all the time and I'm sure they shared needles.

Anyway, because my dad was so messed up on drugs … he would have sex with me and that lasted for a couple of years. I do not remember if he used a condom or not. It was dark and I guess I really didn't know the difference. Anyway, when I found out, I freaked. To make a long story short I got tested in March of this year and it was negative. I didn't tell anyone, not even my mother. I really don't know how I feel about my dad. It's pretty sad because he made such stupid decisions and I don't want him to die." – Anonymous

"Dear Don ... My father had a friend he had known since grade school who shared a needle once and got HIV. His father was a very successful doctor and did everything he could do, but he couldn't save his son. My Dad's friend kept saying, 'All I want to do is live.' But he was stuck with a painful, unfortunate death. A painful death is not worth a moment of fun." – Jordan

"Dear Don ... I especially enjoyed the approach you took to laying out the facts and misconceptions, unlike the DARE program you didn't stand up there and say 'if you do this you will die', instead you laid out the facts for us so that we can now make a decision. I hope you continue speaking with this approach because the DARE approach is so anti-everything that it makes you want to go out and do everything it says not to do just to rebel." – Ted

"Dear Don ... Your talk was very eye opening because as bad as it may seem, I know way too many people that use intravenous drugs. It is not uncommon for one needle to go around to four or five people. I was not aware of the risk of sharing needles and it's kind of scary." – Joe

Prevention: The power of friendship

Not long after I started telling my story to others, a young man in the audience asked, "**Don, what's the worst day you've had in your life, since the first day you learned you had HIV?**" The instant he asked the question, the answer popped into my head. The worst day of my life wasn't the day I learned I had HIV. It wasn't the day I sat in McDonald's in shock as Dennis dropped his pants and urinated on the floor. It wasn't even the day Kenny died, 15 minutes before I showed up at the hospital. **The worst day of my life was the first day I had to change my best friend's diaper.**

I cannot even begin to describe the range of emotions I experienced that day: immense sadness, grief, fear and disbelief. These words only describe part of the feelings, which overwhelmed me that morning as my eyes filled with tears. My best friend, once an independent and brilliant researcher, was now reduced to someone with the mind and capabilities of a small child. How could this have ever happened? How long would it be before someone would be changing my diaper?

Can you imagine yourself changing your best friend's diaper? Or picture your best friend changing yours? I'm sure it's an experience everyone would prefer to avoid.

In this chapter, I've discussed the advantages of abstinence, as well as specific steps you can take to help prevent yourself from contracting HIV. Until now, the chapter has pretty much been all about you protecting yourself. However, there are also some important steps you can take to help ensure your friends and the other people in your life that you love never contract HIV.

Most of us care about the opinions of our friends, more so than those of some of the authority figures in our life (parents, clergy, teachers, etc.). The advice we get from our authority figures often "goes in one ear and out the other." However, most of us tend to take to heart the opinions of our closest friends. If one of our friends tells us we *"screwed up"* or verbally expresses any type of disappointment in our behavior or attitude, we're likely to pay attention.

If you have friends who are putting themselves at risk for HIV, if you care about them, let them know you're worried and explain why. If your friends have a casual outlook about sex, sleep around just for kicks and have a history of multiple partners, ask them to stop. If you have friends who are sexually active with a particular partner, make sure they've had an HIV test and are always practicing safer sex. If you have friends who drink to excess and/or use any drugs, especially IV drugs, make sure they are aware how their behavior is putting them at risk for HIV/AIDS.

Learn to be proactive about protecting yourself and be proactive in helping your friends protect themselves. No one enjoys changing diapers.

Comments: Friends

"Dear Don ... You taught me a lot of new things, like how if you have AIDS you can battle and stay alive. ... The stories you told about your friends impacted the way I look at my friendships. You can't go through this alone and having support of friends and loved ones help so much." – Presley

"Dear Don Carrel ... Seeing you and listening to your story it kind of made me realize that this disease is real and could happen to me or anyone that I know. The thing that really impacted me the most out of your speech though was when you were telling the story about your friend and the accident that happened at McDonald's. I realize it must have been hard for you to talk about, but I am glad that you did because it makes you really understand why you don't want your friends to get the disease." – Brooke

"Dear Don ... I had already planned to abstain from sex, but your presentation gave me all the more reason to wait. I don't think you're crazy, I do believe that your friend did come to you on your front porch and talk to you. Don, you have made me want to talk more with my friends and parents about HIV/AIDS. Your stories are things that need to be heard all over the world. I wish you the best and I pray for you." – Nicole

"Dear Don ... The thing that impacted me the most was the story of how you had to change your best friend's diaper. I was shocked to hear something like that. There's no way I could imagine how that had to feel. I also thought it was really funny when you talked about how your son was telling his friends to always use condoms." – Ethan

"Dear Don ... I had no idea that it was so simple to avoid. I thought that you could just get it from hanging out with someone who has it, but now I know that I can avoid it so easily just by using a condom and not sharing needles, and no oral sex. ... Your story about your friend impacted me a lot. I cannot

believe he died from this disease weighing only 67 pounds. That is so sad and that must have been a really bad loss for you." – Alexis

"Dear Don ... What impacted me during your presentation is the fact that AIDS is one of the most preventable diseases in the world. All you have to do is avoid high-risk behaviors, and you're set. It bothers me to hear that HIV/AIDS is so preventable, yet it is one of the largest pandemics, if not the largest worldwide." – Joseph

"Dear Don Carrel ... Your presentation was the only one all year where I paid attention, and was involved, the entire time. ... I knew a lot about HIV/AIDS, but I wasn't too concerned about it until after I heard your presentation. I've made a promise to myself to not be as risky and really watch myself. I refuse to ruin my future by getting AIDS." – Alison

Comments: "It can't happen to me."

"Dear Don ... I have heard the rhetoric about AIDS before being that it's deadly as well as life debilitating. I think most people get the disease because they say the phrase 'It can't happen to me" over and over again in their head. I'm not immune to AIDS, and you made me realize that." – Love, Danielle

"Dear Don ... It has showed me that sex isn't something to be taken lightly. I had never met anyone I knew with AIDS until you. I had always thought that, 'I'll never get AIDS' or "It could never happen to me' until I met you, an everyday, regular person just like me. I am now more aware that people I see everyday could have AIDS and that person could be someone I may have sex with." – Rachel

"Dear Don ... I had always thought about AIDS, but figured 'It won't happen to me.' After I heard your presentation, it really made me think. I now know how many consequences there could be. It kind of scared me because it's so easy not to get, but yet so easy to get. I now know the precautions I have to take in order not to contract the AIDS virus. You helped everyone realize that AIDS isn't just a little disease, it's one that will change your life forever." – Jackie

Dear Don ... Kids my age need to realize that it can happen to them. I never knew that condoms help reduce the risk of HIV infection. I know people at my school who do use drugs and I don't think they realize it can increase their chances of getting HIV/AIDS." – Kayla

Comments: Prevention

"Dear Don Carrel ... I think that the thing that most impacted me is realizing that I do have a choice to get or not get AIDS. It's not just a random thing, it can be prevented." – Laura

"Dear Don ... Your speech really opened up my eyes. If our class had read it out of a book or watched some movie about AIDS, I would have forgotten the information already, but learning about it through you was <u>so real</u>. I think that because you came to our class, I will have a slimmer chance of getting AIDS because I know what to do to prevent it." – Zach

"Don ... It scares me to think of how many people are dying from a disease that can be prevented. It scares me even more to know that one of my friends could have HIV and not know it. I'm not at risk because I'm abstinent and drug-free. I wish more people would get tested for the disease and at least think twice before having unprotected sex with a one-night stand or sharing IV needles." – Julie

"Dear Mr. Don Carrel ... I respect how you understand that all teens are not abstinent, so giving tips about how to use condoms and getting an HIV test were very helpful." – Sara

"Dear Don ... Thank you for telling us about the girl who told you about how she and her boyfriend always use a condom and get tested for HIV every 6 months. That is something. When I become sexually active (which I'm not yet and don't plan to be for a long while) I plan to do the same. ... Thank you for making me realize how bad this disease really is and how it can affect a person." – Amy

"Dear Don ... I'm sure your message got across to everyone there to either practice safer sex or abstinence." – JP

"Dear Don ... I don't know about everyone else, but I definitely got the picture that AIDS is a very serious subject and is not to be taken lightly. I also know now that it's a disease that I or anyone else on this planet does not have to get." – Josh

"Mr. Carrel ... I believe it is incredibly important that both the young and the old learn about the detrimental effects of the HIV virus and AIDS." – Ashley

Conclusion

According to the Kaiser Family Foundation, the U.S. federal funding for HIV in 2010 was $26 billion, which equals approximately $86 for each American. Of this $26 billion, 62 percent was allocated to help care for HIV/AIDS patients (medication, housing assistance, etc.), 11 percent was used for research, 25 percent was spent for programs to help with the international pandemic and only 3 percent was used for HIV prevention programs.

The good news: During the last decade, HIV infection rates have decreased approximately 20 percent worldwide. The bad news: During the last decade, HIV infection rates in the United States have **not decreased** 20 percent. In fact, over the last decade the HIV infection rates in the U.S. have **increased.** According to the Centers for Disease Control, more than 56,000 Americans are newly infected with HIV every year. In 1990, approximately 500,000 Americans were living with HIV/AIDS. Today, the number of Americans living with HIV/AIDS is possibly three times higher than the number living with the disease 20 years ago, and that number is continuing to increase every year. Today, approximately one out of every 160 Americans between the ages of 15 and 59 has HIV/AIDS.

Since beginning my personal crusade to help others avoid HIV infection, I've become increasingly infuriated by the fact that our federal government has never taken an aggressive role in preventing its citizens from becoming another AIDS statistic. Allocating only 3 percent of the federal HIV budget for prevention is pathetic. Does it not make sense to do everything possible to lower the number of Americans who may become infected with HIV? Additional funding for programs to prevent individuals from contracting HIV would obviously be less expensive than providing care to those who become infected simply because they're not sufficiently educated about how easy it is to prevent. As individuals and as a nation, we must do more to stop the spread of this dreadful disease.

"Dear Don ... I believe the media downplays HIV/AIDS so much, especially in the United States. Many people just believe that AIDS is only something that is spread in Third World countries such as Africa. But the reality is that it happens in the U.S. too, and students are not being taught anything about prevention."
– Angela

There is currently no cure for AIDS, and no cure or vaccine is expected anytime soon. Medical treatment for those with HIV/AIDS has improved dramatically, making HIV/AIDS more of a chronic illness rather than a fatal disease. However, comprehensive treatment is unbelievably expensive and is out of the reach of many of those infected.

Prevention is still the best weapon we have to fight the HIV/AIDS epidemic.

Epilogue

A few months back, I ran across a description of "life with HIV" posted to a blog by Richard S. Ferri, PhD., a writer who also happens to be an HIV nurse practitioner. The post: *"Living with HIV is never just about one virus. Living with HIV is about your life being twisted like two cars in a head on collision. Some of us are lucky and able to extract ourselves from the wreckage and get on with our lives; others never do."*

Ferri summed up in three short sentences my life with HIV. Years ago, when I first suspected I might be HIV-positive, when I realized I was about to have a *head-on collision* my thoughts were somewhere between disbelief and terror. When I was finally tested for HIV, the *collision* occurred. I went into shock and had no idea if I would survive the initial impact. I spent months struggling to *extract myself from the wreckage.* I had to make a choice – *get on with my life* – or die.

I chose to live. Even as my friends were getting sick and dying, I chose to live. I refused to get sick. I had two sons to support. Every night before going to sleep, my prayers included a simple request: *"Please, God, let me feel as good tomorrow as I feel today."* That simple prayer was answered for many years.

Since contracting HIV, I've learned to look at my glass of life as half full, rather than half empty. Having HIV has helped me understand that life is a journey. A journey with more obstacles for some than others, but a journey we all have the ability to enjoy regardless of our personal trials and tribulations.

"Dear Don … Your speech really made me realize how precious life really is. People need to live each day to the fullest, because no one ever knows when or how they will die. I admire you so much for the dedication you put into stopping the spread of this disease. To me, you are the true definition of a hero." – Erica

"Dear Don ... First off, I would like to thank you for devoting your time to speak to our class. It takes one heck of a person to have the strength to do what you do. You are what no text-book or pamphlet could be. You took us into your life. Secondly, I would like to tell you how I felt about your talk with us. I found it greatly inspiring. I don't know how many people may react to your presentations, but I was totally swept away. Everything that you talked about was a lesson in human behavior and adjustment. I certainly look up to you for your courage and strength. There are people out there that would just decide life isn't worth living if you know you are going to die sometime in the near future. That's just the wrong attitude, and you are the exact opposite from that. Thank you again." – Kevin

"Dear Don ... The quote that was the most mind boggling was, 'When you have AIDS, dying isn't the hard part.' It's a terrible death that one has to live with. But that's exactly what occurs and although you have a horrible death, one can still have an incredible life. You're not dying, you are living a brilliantly vibrant life and that is the greatest thing I learned." – Love, Danielle

In the first chapter of this book, I wrote, "Having HIV is a huge **blessing** in my life." You may have found my statement difficult to comprehend. Hopefully, while reading this book, you've picked up on some of the many reasons I truly feel fortunate to have been infected with HIV.

Of my many blessings, there are two in particular that have greatly enriched my life. One of the two involves a dramatic change in how I view myself. The other involves the change and growth in my personal faith – in my belief in God.

The directive given to me by "the messenger" during a dream in 1995 changed the course of my life. By doing nothing more than sharing my story with others, I've been blessed with the ability to touch many lives. I have been privileged with the opportunity to change thoughts, attitudes and hopefully the behavior of thousands of teens and young adults. In turn, those who listened to my story have had an enormous impact on my pilgrimage to learn to love myself.

A number of years ago, I was in the locker room at the gym changing shoes when a young man approached me. He looked at me and tentatively inquired, *"You're Don aren't you?"* Stopping mid-stream while tying my shoe, I looked up, smiled and replied, *"Yes, I'm Don."* He continued the conversation, *"I thought it was* *you. You don't know me, but I want to thank you. I just graduated from KU. I heard you speak six years ago when I was in high school at Shawnee Mission East. I want you to know that because of <u>you</u> – I have <u>never</u> had sex without a condom."*

Upon hearing those words, I instantly felt warm and fuzzy, as if I were encompassed in a huge, loving embrace – an embrace from "the messenger." I choked up and my eyes swelled with tears as I smiled at the young man and thanked him for his message.

Exhilarated, I drove home thinking to myself, *"I've spent thousands of hours teaching others how to protect themselves from HIV. My one brief encounter this morning, and the 'thank you' I received, more than 'paid' me for many years of effort."*

I have been blessed with an opportunity to save lives. Before I ever meet with any group, I always pray silently that no one hearing my story on that day will ever contract HIV. I pray for the ability to deliver a message that will, in some way, impact each and every person's desire to protect not only themselves, but also their friends and family from this dreadful disease.

"Don ... On a personal note, I truly respect your personality and purpose. Your personality because during the time you spoke to us you had a smile on your face as if, even through the worst circumstances, you still enjoy life. Your purpose because you have spent your valuable time to save lives, which is more than most in this world, could say. I wish only the best for you in the many decades you will live on." – Tyler

"Dear Mr. Carrel ... I speak on behalf of my fellow classmates and myself when I say that we truly appreciate you coming in to speak with us. Not only is it a brave thing that you do, it is also empowering. I am glad you are choosing to inform teens and others of this disease, because many people think they are immortal and the truth is it can happen to anyone. .... You are a blessing, a messenger from God, and what you are doing is not in vain. Though you are only one person, you are changing thousands of people's lives and I thank you for that. May you be blessed Mr. Don." – Diamond

Over the years, it has become increasingly apparent that while I'm effectively teaching others why and how to protect themselves from HIV, I'm inadvertently teaching them something perhaps even more important, that life is precious and should be both valued and enjoyed.

"Dear Don ... After you talked to my class last week, I started thinking about what part of the speech impacted me the most. It wasn't really the technical stuff but more the big picture. I guess I never realized that the problems I face every day don't even compare to the daily struggle of people with AIDS. I now look at life as more than tomorrow. I'm not sure that it makes sense, but I want to live every day to the fullest." – Jeff

"Dear Don ... I have never really thought about life. Life is something that sometimes you don't think about until you have been confronted with something that can change it. HIV/AIDS is something that can change your life by making only one mistake. That's what I have learned from you during your presentation. I really thought about how precious life can be. I think you are such a brave person to fight and never give up." – Perri

"Dear Don ... As I walked into the classroom the first person I saw was you. You looked me right in the eye as I walked to my seat in the front row. You looked so strong and proud and your courage amazed me. Your presentation hit me hard and there were times I just wanted to hug you. When I left class I started crying. I want to thank you for going on each day and for teaching us what we need to know." – Teegan

"Dear Don ... The world needs more people like you. You are so courageous, honest, compassionate and a thousand other things. What you are doing and how you've survived is really inspirational. I know that your speech also impacted my classmates. I often heard remarks in the halls about how brave your were. I can't thank you enough for what you've done for so many people. You are truly a hero. All my Love and Best of Luck" Jenny

"Hero, brave, courageous, honest, compassionate, strong, proud, inspiring" are all words that have be used to describe me in letters I have received from hundreds of people.

It appears as if I've been blessed with the ability to influence others, not so much because of what I say, but because of who I am.

The doubts about my self-esteem that I harbored starting early in my childhood and carried throughout most of my adult life are gone. By embracing "the messenger's" wish, I've experienced the joy that comes from helping others. I've learned that the true recipients of the time and resources exerted by volunteers are the volunteers themselves. When you give of yourself to help others, you are repaid for your efforts many times over.

Talking about my life with HIV/AIDS has resulted in my learning to love myself, which is something I'm not sure would have ever happened had my life's journey been any different.

In addition to learning to love myself, living with HIV and AIDS has had a profound effect on my faith. Hundreds, if not thousands of times, I've been asked if I believe in God.

As a child, I was raised in a "C and E" Christian household – one where attending church on Christmas and Easter was automatic, but throughout the rest of the year attendance was sporadic. As I matured, I wasn't necessarily a nonbeliever, but by no means was I convinced that God existed.

When Karen and I started dating in college, she was Catholic, so I began to attend Mass with her weekly. Her parents, Ralph and Barb, were devout Catholics, and I admired their strong faith and the impact it had on their relationship over the years. Before graduating from college, I made the decision to convert to Catholicism. Karen and I were married in the church and I attended Mass weekly until our divorce.

Once divorced, I agreed to go through the necessary procedure to have our marriage annulled to allow Karen to remarry in the Catholic Church. It was my understanding that annulments were automatically granted if a marriage had never been consummated or if the husband or wife happened to be gay or lesbian.

Since I didn't come to grips with my sexual orientation until after my marriage, I assumed getting an annulment would be as simple as acknowledging the fact I was gay. Without going into detail, my annulment experience soured my attitude not only about the Catholic Church, but also my view of "organized" religion. My life as a practicing Catholic came to an end.

Several years later, I made the decision to give organized religion another chance. I joined a Christian church in Manhattan, Kansas, where many people affiliated with Manhattan Christian College (MCC) worshipped. My partner at the time, Damon, had graduated from MCC and was a worship leader, Sunday school teacher and in line to become a deacon in the church. When I made the decision to join, I was re-baptized by full immersion in front of the entire congregation, an experience I didn't take lightly. For the next few months, Damon and I attended services together and were warmly received and welcomed by everyone. However, once someone discovered that our relationship was closer than that of "roommates," the news spread like wildfire. We arrived one Sunday morning for the service and were shunned by the entire congregation.

If you check the dictionary for the word "shun," you'll find the following definition: to avoid, evade, steer clear of, shy away from, keep one's distance from, have nothing to do with: snub, give someone the cold shoulder, ignore, look right through, etc. Yes, the entire congregation completely ignored us, refused to even acknowledge our *"hellos"* and literally pretended we weren't there. Embarrassed, hurt and angry, I asked myself, *"How can these people call themselves Christians?"*

A few days later the church elders paid a visit to our home to inform Damon they did not approve of our lifestyle and he had been removed from his positions at the church. My life as a church-going Christian came to an abrupt end.

My nearly back-to-back experiences with first the Catholic Church and then a fundamentalist Christian church destroyed my belief in organized religion for many years. That being said, I was aware at the time, and still understand today, that many of the views held by members of religious organizations are determined by humans and not by the power that created our universe.

My personal discovery of faith did not actually begin until the day I picked up my HIV test results from Dr. Wade, the day I was told to get my affairs in order because the odds were I had only two years to live. Driving home that day, I prayed desperately for not two years of life, but for 10, to live long enough to get Chris and Matt out of high school.

My prayer on that day was the first time in my life that I sincerely asked, actually begged, God for help. I repeated this prayer once or twice daily, for the next 10 years. During the first two or three years as I was reaching out to God in prayer, I watched a number of my friends physically deteriorate and finally die from complications of AIDS. Yet, I continued to remain healthy. As the years passed, with my health stable, I slowly began to believe that God truly existed and was answering my prayer.

When Dennis finally succumbed to AIDS and I lost my best friend, I found a huge void in my life. I missed him immensely. The emptiness I felt filled to a great extent several years later, when Dennis "returned" for his brief visit, told me he was okay, that everything was wonderful and that I had nothing to fear. On that day, I became a true believer in God.

Not that I needed any further proof about the existence of God, but five years later, while on my deathbed, I had a dream. A dream in which "the messenger" informed me that I would be starting a journey and focus on helping others. A journey where I learned to put my fate into the hands of God.

As someone who has been face-to-face with death, I've often reflected on the miracle of life. It's impossible for me to even begin to comprehend the magnitude of the force that was necessary to create our universe, and the intellect required to design not only mankind but also all the simpler life forms on earth.

Yes, I believe in God. All of us have different visions of God based on what we've learned from our family, church and personal experiences.

My vision of God is too grand to describe simply as an old white-headed man perched on a throne. It's difficult for me to believe that one being, in human form, possesses the power or vision to have created our universe and everything in it.

I personally imagine God to be a vast expanse of power which surrounds and flows through everything, including every one of us. I believe we all have the choice to recognize the power of God within us, and use that power to make the world a better place.

As a child, my grandmother often repeated the Golden Rule to me: *"Do unto others as you would have them do unto you."* The Golden Rule has a long history and has been repeated in one form or another by religious figures and philosophers since the beginning of ancient civilization. Some version of this basic concept of human rights exists in almost every religion known to mankind, yet it has often been ignored in the name of specific religious beliefs. I genuinely believe that religious opinions that seek to circumvent the simplicity of the Golden Rule came about and continue to evolve based on the thoughts of individuals and are not part of God's plan.

I now have a church home, Unity, which shares a vision of God very similar to my own. God as a magnificent power – where the focus is on loving one another and treating others in the way we would all like to be treated. I have a church home where judging others is not part of the teachings.

If all mankind embraced and followed the Golden Rule, there would be no hate, no wars and our world would be, as my friend Dennis would say, "a wonderful place."

Acknowledgments

To "the messenger," thank you for starting me on an incredible journey. Thank you for the ability to share my story passionately and for the strength to finish this book, which hopefully will continue to protect others from HIV/AIDS long after I'm gone.

To Chris Curry, my partner and #1 editor, thank you for spending nearly as many hours proofing my work as I did writing it. I'm grateful for your wisdom in "suggesting" that I hire another editor to take a more objective look at my writing. Even more than your grammar skills, thank you for your never-ending emotional support, encouragement and love.

To Lisbeth Tanz, my #2 editor and new good friend, thank you for helping me (aka "Ernie" Hemingway) learn to put the emotion I feel into words that express those emotions. Thank you for not allowing me to put dashes – in every sentence. Thank you for not "losing it" every time "Ernie" emailed you an addition or change to chapters he had already submitted as finished. Thank you for being "kind" when saying, *"I'm sorry Ernie, but you have to take that part out … it doesn't belong in your book."* Thank you for your genuine belief that my story is one that should be heard by everyone. I'm thankful that my good friend, Annie Sorensen, recommended you as my editor. www.yourwordsyourvoice.com.

To Kevin Garrison, thank you for donating your time, talent and patience, especially your patience, in transforming my book cover concept into a colorful, whimsical design that perfectly reflects my vision.

To Chris Porter, thank you for bravely and eloquently sharing your story as part of this book. I'm thankful for our shared desire to prevent others from living life with HIV/AIDS.

To my son, Chris Carrel, thank you for donating your technical skills to create the *"My Dream to Trample AIDS"* website: www.TrampleAIDS.com.

To Peggy Rose, thank you for being one of the first educators who allowed me the chance to tell my story to teenagers and for sharing your thoughts in the foreword of this book.

To Sue Chipman, thank you for your friendship and for providing your testimony for my book cover. Thank you for the opportunity to share my story with every one of your health students since 1996.

Thank you to Sue Storm, Nancy McRoberts, Carla Vause and Christi Posey for their kind comments included on the book flap of the hardcover edition of *My Dream to Trample AIDS.*

Thank you to the thousands of teenagers and young adults who have taken the time to write to me over the years to express their appreciation and share their own stories. I'm especially grateful to those whose comments are included in this book.

To Matthew Murry of Dog Ear Publishing, thank you for assisting this first-time author in the publication of *My Dream to Trample AIDS.*

To my many friends and family members, thank you for your constant love and support. I also would like to say a special *"thank you"* to those of you who allowed me to include your thoughts as part of my written story. And another special *"thank you"* to those of you who helped re-read thousands of letters from students, proofread or in any other way helped in the creation of this book.

To the readers of this book, thank you for taking the time to read my story. I would appreciate your help in slowing the spread of HIV/AIDS. Please help by recommending this book to your friends, family and acquaintances. I would greatly appreciate any comments you would like to share. You can contact me by going to the *My Dream to Trample AIDS* website **www.TrampleAIDS.com** and sending me a message.

Author Disclaimer

In writing this book, I attempted to provide accurate information for the readers. It is my hope that by reading the material contained in this book people will learn how to substantially reduce their risk of HIV infection. However, statements or ideas suggested should not be construed as medical or professional advice.

As I mentioned in the book, there's no such thing as "safe sex." I've suggested possible ways to reduce the risk of infection of HIV and other STDs by applying "safer sex" suggestions. Anyone acting on ideas or recommendations in the book does so at his or her own risk.

Hopefully, the readers will find the contents of this book helpful and useful. However, I do not guarantee the reliability or accuracy of any of the statistical information, advice or other information contained in this book. In addition, I cannot guarantee the material obtained from any website, book, newspaper or magazine referenced in this book is accurate. I do not warrant the authenticity of any links or websites mentioned.

The entire contents of this book are provided for educational purposes only. I disclaim all warranties of any kind, whether expressed or implied.

Carrel Care, LLC, © copyrights this book. No part of this book may be copied, sold or used in any way without written permission from the author.

Author contact information may found at: **www.TrampleAIDS.com.**

About the Author

Don Carrel has been living with AIDS since 1995. He suspects he was infected with HIV in 1981. Thirty years later, less than 2 percent of people with HIV have lived long enough to share their stories. In 1995, while lying in a hospital bed with Pneumocystis pneumonia, the most common form of death for someone with AIDS, Don had a riveting dream that dramatically altered his life and, perhaps the future lives of more than 100,000 teenagers. After making a full recovery, Don set out to teach young people what they needed to know about HIV prevention so that they wouldn't wind up in his shoes. His lofty goal: to stomp out AIDS. After 16 years, Don has collected thousands of thank-you letters from teens and adults who have heard his compelling presentations. Today, Don hopes to reach an even wider audience with his book, *My Dream to Trample AIDS*.

Don grew up in Shawnee, Kansas, a suburb of Kansas City. He graduated from Shawnee Mission North High School and attended Kansas State University in Manhattan, Kansas, where he earned a bachelor's degree in business management. While at K-State, he met Karen, whom he married. They had two sons, Christopher and Matthew.

During the first 10 years of his career, Don built a successful insurance and investment business. At 23, he was one of the youngest members ever inducted into the Million Dollar Roundtable.

In 1982, Don changed careers to pursue another passion. He opened a gourmet-gift shop in Manhattan called *Kitchens Plus* and a restaurant, *The Croissant Café*, which served fresh-baked pastries, lunch and homemade desserts to several hundred shoppers every day.

In 1991, Don moved back to the Kansas City area and a few years later opened a store called *Kids Plus Me*. This original retail concept specialized in toys for children of all ages and also carried a unique selection of products especially chosen for "Mom," who typically was the one shopping for toys for her children.

As part of his volunteer work of educating others about HIV prevention, in 2000, Don decided to form a team of young people to walk with him in the annual AIDS Walk Kansas City. More than 1,500 students showed up to support Don — possibly the largest AIDS Walk team in history. In three years, his group, *Don's Teens Trample AIDS,* raised more than $100,000 to help those suffering from HIV/AIDS.

For his tireless volunteer efforts in HIV education as well as fundraising in the Kansas City area, the AIDS Service Foundation of Greater Kansas City awarded Don a prestigious Ribbon of Hope award in 2005.

Don currently resides in Mission, Kansas, with his partner, Chris, and their dogs, Ellie and Emma. He continues to speak whenever he is asked to share his message to prevent HIV — and ultimately his dream to trample AIDS.

Index

CPSIA information can be obtained at www.ICGtesting.com
Printed in the USA
LVOW081842141111

254973LV00003B/1/P